Praise for *Food Science for Gardeners*

If you eat what you grow, you need this book! Robert Pavlis' *Food Science for Gardeners* will absolutely help any gardener grow nutritionally dense food. He not only expertly teaches the necessary science, but how to apply it for the best results.

—Jeff Lowenfels, a.k.a. Lord of the Roots, and author, *Teaming With Microbes* Tetralogy and *DIY Autoflowering Cannabis*

With *Food Science for Gardeners*, Robert Pavlis had written another essential guide, this time presenting the kind of information on growing and preserving safe, healthy, and nutritious food that isn't found in gardening books. Up-to-date, scientific, and leavened with common sense, what a useful reference this is for anyone interested in growing food!

—Linda Gilkeson, educator and author, *Backyard Bounty*

This is a much needed book! We need to get back to nature and the food that keeps us healthy. Learning to grow food is easy and enjoyable with just a little bit of knowledge. Roll up your sleeves and let this amazing book get you started on your journey to great health and a fun garden!

—Lynn Gillespie, organic farmer, thelivingfarm.org

Praise for Robert Pavlis and the Garden Science series

I've been following Robert's work for a long time and I trust his science-based, no-nonsense approach to helping us all debunk gardening myths while making us all smarter gardeners in the process. Robert is one of my trusted, go-to sources when I want to get to the bottom line.

—Joe Lamp'l, Creator and Host of Emmy Award-winning PBS television series, *Growing a Greener World*® and Founder, joegardener.com and The joe gardener® Show podcast

It's hard not to appreciate Pavlis' clear and consistently myth-busting approach, guiding the reader with a precise balance of science and analogy. There is loads of good information coupled with actionable insight throughout.

—Jesse Frost, author, *The Living Soil Handbook: The No-till Grower's Guide to Ecological Market Gardening*

Robert Pavlis has provided another detailed, yet accessible, addition to gardeners' home libraries. Be sure to give *Plant Science for Gardeners* an honored place on your bookshelves, next to Mr. Pavlis' groundbreaking *Garden Myths* series.

—Rebecca Martin, technical editor, *Mother Earth News* magazine

food science for gardeners

food science for gardeners

Grow, Harvest, and Prepare Nutrient-Dense Food

ROBERT PAVLIS

new society PUBLISHERS

Cover design by Diane McIntosh.
Cover image: © iStock (#1307632045)
Page 1: © 399715431 / Adobe Stock

Printed in Canada. First printing September 2024.

Any other inquiries can be directed by mail to:

New Society Publishers
P.O. Box 189, Gabriola Island, BC V0R 1X0, Canada
(250) 247-9737

LIBRARY AND ARCHIVES CANADA CATALOGUING IN PUBLICATION

Title: Food science for gardeners : grow, harvest, and prepare nutrient dense foods / Robert Pavlis.

Names: Pavlis, Robert, author

Description: Series statement: Garden science series ; 5 | Includes bibliographical references and index.

Identifiers: Canadiana (print) 20240437950 | Canadiana (ebook) 20240437977 | ISBN 9780865719781 (softcover) | ISBN 9781550927726 (PDF) | ISBN 9781771423687 (EPUB)

Subjects: LCSH: Vegetables. | LCSH: Vegetable gardening. | LCSH: Plant nutrients. | LCSH: Nutrition. | LCSH: Food—Safety measures. | LCSH: Food science.

Classification: LCC SB320.9 .P38 2024 | DDC 63—dc23

Funded by the Government of Canada | Financé par le gouvernement du Canada | Canada

New Society Publishers' mission is to publish books that contribute in fundamental ways to building an ecologically sustainable and just society, and to do so with the least possible impact on the environment, in a manner that models this vision.

new society PUBLISHERS

Certified B Corporation

FSC www.fsc.org MIX Paper | Supporting responsible forestry FSC® C016245

Contents

1. Introduction 3
Why Do We Eat? 3
What Is Food Quality? 5
Do Gardeners Produce High Quality Food? 6
Gardeners Affect Quality 7
The History of Food Science 9

2. Understanding Nutrition 11
Human Nutrients vs Plant Nutrients 12
Nutrients vs Calories 13
Nutrients in Food 14
Factors Affecting Nutrients 29
Nutrition Myths 31

3. Food Safety—Chemicals 33
Chemical Toxicity 35
Pesticides 38
Heavy Metals 41
Food Safe Plastics 45
Safe Material for Raised Beds 48
Microplastics 51
Growing Food Near Toxic Plants 51
Allelopathy 52
GMO Food 53
Allergies and Sensitivities 56

4. Food Safety—Biological 59
The Microbes Among Us 60
What Is a Foodborne Illness 61
How Microbes Grow 63
Detecting a Problem 68

Buying Food 70
Food Safety Myths 70
Final Thoughts 74

5. Nutrient Density 75
Measuring Nutrient Density 76
Factors Affecting Nutrient Density 80
What Does Science Know About Growing Nutrient-Dense Food? 83
Factors Affecting Nutrients 86

6. The Flavor of Food 89
Nutrition and Flavor 94
Why Does Grocery Store Produce Taste Bland? 96
Sweetness vs Acidity 97
Factors Affecting Flavor 98

7. Growing Great Food 105
Selecting the Right Cultivar 106
Importance of Days to Maturity 107
Heirlooms vs Hybrids 108
Is Organic Food Better? 114
Fresh Is Best 118

8. Handling and Storing Food 125
Washing Hands and Produce 125
Food Storage 130

9. Preserving Food 135
Preserving Techniques 135
Methods for Preserving Food 137

10. Cooking Food 159
Why Do We Cook Food? 159
How Does Cooking Affect Flavor? 161
How Does Cooking Affect Nutrition?. 164
Cooking Creates Undesirable Compounds 165
Food That Needs Cooking 169
Cooking Myths 172
Cooking Methods 172

11. **Growing and Serving Quality Food** 181
Beans, Green (Snap Beans) 181
Cucumbers 182
Garlic 183
Lettuce 184
Onion 185
Peas 186
Radish 186
Raspberries 187
Strawberries 188
Tomato 189
Zucchini 190

Notes 191

Index 197

About the Author 205

Connect with Robert Pavlis 207

About New Society Publishers 214

Famous quote:
"If you can't pronounce it, don't eat it."
Attributed to "Nonsense"

This popular belief is wrong, as you will see in this book. Many of the healthy "chemicals" in food are unpronounceable. Take for example the contents of a natural healthy banana:

Ingredients: Water (75%), Sugars (12%) (Glucose (48%), Fructose (40%), Sucrose (2%), Maltose (<1%)), Starch (5%), Fibre E460 (3%), Amino Acids (<1%) (Glutamic Acid (19%), Aspartic Acid (16%), Histidine (11%), Leucine (7%), Lysine (5%), Phenylalanine (4%), Arginine (4%), Valine (4%), Alanine (4%), Serine (4%), Glycine (3%), Threonine (3%), Isoleucine (3%), Proline (3%), Tryptophan (1%), Cystine (1%), Tyrosine (1%), Methionine (1%)), Fatty Acids (1%) (Palmitic Acid (30%), Omega-6 Fatty Acid: Linoleic Acid (14%), Omega-3 Fatty Acid: Linolenic Acid (8%), Oleic Acid (7%), Palmitoleic Acid (3%), Stearic Acid (2%), Lauric Acid (1%), Myristic Acid (1%), Capric Acid (<1%)), Ash (<1%), Phytosterols, E515, Oxalic Acid, E300, E306 (Tocopherol), Phylloquinone, Thiamin, Colours (Yellow-Orange E101 (Riboflavin), Yellow-Brown E160a), Flavours (3-Methylbut-1-Yl Ethanoate, 2-Methylbutyl Ethanoate, 2-Methylpropan-1-Ol, 3-Methylbutyl-1-Ol, 2- Hydroxy-3-Methylethyl Butanoate, 3-Methylbutanal, Ethyl Hexanoate, Ethyl Butanoate, Pentyl Acetate), 1510, Natural Ripening Agent (Ethene Gas).

Credit: James Kennedy, Melbourne, Australia (Tianjinren88)

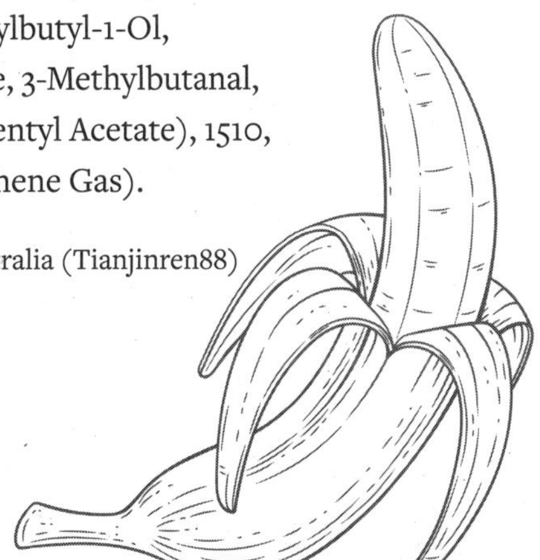

1
Introduction

Food science is the study of food and how it affects our health. It combines several disciplines including chemistry, biochemistry, nutrition, microbiology, and engineering to solve problems associated with the food system. Food science looks at the basic chemical components of food and tries to understand how they are affected by various preserving and processing techniques, such as freezing, drying, pasteurizing, dehydrating, and canning. It then looks at how all of this affects our health with a focus on nutrition.

As a gardener, you have a special connection with food science. You not only care about the food you buy but also the food you grow. In fact, many of you are growing food to ensure that you have access to the most nutritious food possible. This book bridges the divide between nutrition and gardening. It will provide the background needed to fully understand the nutritional value of food and then show you how your activities in the garden and the kitchen can improve the quality of your food.

Why Do We Eat?

On a very basic level, we eat because we are hungry, but why are we hungry? After a meal, our gastrointestinal tract slowly empties by pushing food through the stomach, then the small intestine, and finally the large intestine. This process is regulated by hormones that also cause the rumbling in our stomach and the activation of specific neurons in our brain, signaling us that it's time to eat again.

The digestion process takes about two hours, which explains why we crave a snack between meals. Appetite is simply the desire to eat. It can be due to hunger, but many times it has other causes such as feeling stressed, upset, bored, or being exposed to food that looks or smells delicious. How do you tell if it is hunger or appetite? Select a healthy food you don't hate but don't particularly enjoy. If you eat it, you were probably hungry.

We also eat for pleasure. Nobody needs a glass of wine or a chocolate brownie after dinner. We eat these because we enjoy them. Since we have a huge selection of different food sources and many ways to prepare them, we also tend to eat things we like.

We eat with our eyes. How food looks is almost as important as how it tastes, but taste is critical and we use it to make food choices. Broccoli looks great and is good for you, but you only eat it if you like the taste—or if your mother makes you eat it!

Our taste preferences are present when we are born and even babies prefer sweets and fats. As babies mature, they develop a palate for other flavors. Studies have shown that children who are exposed to a wide variety of food are more likely to enjoy a wide range of flavors as adults.

On a biological level, we eat to stay alive. Our body needs a continuous supply of nutrients in order to function and to provide enough energy to carry out all of our internal processes. Our bodies are like factories. We need a constant supply of raw materials (the nutrients) that get turned into products such as hair, skin, blood cells, antibodies, and proteins. Factories also need a source of energy to make everything happen, and our bodies are no different.

A healthy diet includes all of the required nutrients and a good energy supply, but there is another aspect to consider. A diet is only healthy if it also excludes harmful elements such as carcinogens and toxic chemicals. Understanding these aspects of food is critical for gardeners since their actions in the garden directly affect the contents of food.

What Is Food Quality?

There are a lot of discussions about food quality. Is spinach better than green beans? Berries are rich in antioxidants, but does that make them better than other food? Are animals a better source of protein than vegetables? Some foods have a high nutrient density, while corn is just empty calories. Are these statements even correct? What does all this mean, and how do we measure food quality?

The definition for food quality is very squishy, meaning that it is not well defined. You won't find a "Food Quality Number" stamped on any food item. In general terms, it is the sum of all properties and attributes of a food item that are of value to the consumer. It includes some obvious attributes such as texture, taste, flavor, appearance, and nutritional content, but it also includes things such as sustainable production, origin, type of production (organic vs non-organic) and safety characteristics.

Food quality is very much a personal opinion. The importance of the above characteristics vary from person to person. For some, price is a major factor, while for others, the fact that it is grown organically is of prime importance.

Since we eat to stay alive and remain healthy you might think that nutrition is most important, but it rarely is. When was the last time you saw a nutritional breakdown for a tomato or a chicken breast? As shoppers we have no idea which fresh food is of higher nutritional value and many times we put our trust in brands.

Most countries have a government organization responsible for setting and enforcing food safety standards and they might also regulate the labels on manufactured food, but few try to regulate other forms of quality. Food manufacturing companies also have standards that they follow, but each company defines their own "quality" standards. For the most part, it is up to individuals to set their own quality standards and unfortunately you are given very little data to use for your decisions. Face it, for the most part you are flying blind when it comes to selecting quality food, especially unprocessed food. Hopefully this book will help you make more informed decisions.

Do Gardeners Produce High Quality Food?

One of the main reasons gardeners grow their own food is to get the highest quality food possible, but does that really happen?

You can't beat the freshness of your homegrown food. There is nothing like going into the garden and eating a ripe tomato right off the vine. Even if you are going to cook the food, you can pick it just before you start making your meal.

Taste is another good reason for growing your own. You can select the cultivars you like best and pick them when they are perfectly ripe. This does mean that you have to visit the garden almost daily. Skip a few days and that perfect pea or bean is now overripe and starting to get woody. Even if you don't pick it at exactly the perfect time, it is usually better than store-bought produce.

What about nutrition? How do the nutrients in homegrown food compare to commercial food? I have never met a gardener who had their homegrown produce tested, so gardeners don't really know how nutritious their food is. As you will see in this book, appearance and taste have very little to do with nutrition.

Food tends to have the highest nutrient level at the time it is picked, provided it is picked at a ripe stage. Some nutrients start deteriorating soon after picking. Vitamins and antioxidants in some types of imported produce may be 100 percent lower than local crops simply due to shipping time. North American grown produce takes about five days to get from the farm to the store. Food from outside of North America can be in transit for a couple of weeks. Add to this a couple of days in the store and in your fridge before you finally eat it.

Based on these facts one would expect that local food is always more nutritious, but there is a catch. Not all nutrients deteriorate as quickly as the abovementioned ones. The quantity of many of the nutrients are just as high in imported produce as compared to locally grown. As you will see later in the book, we don't really have a good way to quantify "total nutrition," and therefore it is not really correct to say one food is more nutritious than another. We can, however, compare two food items for a particular nutrient, or even a list of nutrients.

One of the issues with growing your own food is that a particular food item is only available for a short period of time. A solution to this is to either store the food or process it so that it keeps for a longer period of time. For example, you can grow potatoes and then store them in a root cellar until needed. Or you can make pickles out of your fresh cucumbers.

Is such locally grown preserved food more nutritious than the same food imported from a part of the world that is harvesting fresh produce? What about food that is growing under glass in hydroponics? Is that food as nutritious as homegrown preserved food? The answers are complicated. In many cases, the fresh produce has a higher nutritional content since nutrients are lost during processing. So although local food is more nutritious if eaten fresh, it may be less nutritious than other options when it is consumed out of season.

Gardeners would argue that their own food has a much higher quality to start with and that they control any added chemicals. This is quite true and may mean that your own preserved food is more nutritious than fresh imports.

This whole topic is much more complicated than people realize. For example, it is quite common to see a statement similar to this: "Evidence shows that locally grown produce can have a higher nutritional value than produce transported long distances. Studies have shown that the vitamin C found in local oranges contains more vitamin C than imported oranges." The problem with such a statement is that only one nutrient has been measured and there is no data on any of the other thousands of nutrients. Unless all of them are measured it is incorrect to conclude that one option is more nutritious than another. We will have a deeper dive into this topic in the next chapter.

Gardeners Affect Quality

You have limited options when you buy food at a supermarket. In my store we have regular bananas and organic bananas, and nobody knows where either one came from or how they were grown. We have two types of red peppers; field grown and grown in a greenhouse. The field grown are riper but not always in great condition. The ones grown in a greenhouse are a bit underripe. I have no idea how either is grown.

One of the advantages of growing your own food is that you know exactly how it was grown. You know the cultivar, the soil you used, how you fertilized the plants, and when you watered them. You have the power to do everything right to produce the best possible product—or do you?

One of the problems with backyard gardeners is that they do very little if any testing. They don't match fertilizer levels to plant needs. In many cases they don't even apply the nutrients in appropriate amounts to match their specific soil, and soil improvements are ad hoc at best. Some compost is added yearly, but the quality of the compost is not quantified. A big problem with raised beds is that they tend to have such high levels of phosphate that they actually stunt plant growth. All of these things affect the quality of the food produced.

The harvested produce is not tested for nutrition. It tastes good and it is fresh, but the gardener has no way to quantify the quality of the food. This isn't necessarily a problem, but it is important for all gardeners to understand that every decision they make in the garden has some effect on the quality of the food they produce. When it comes to fruits and vegetables, it is not just about getting a harvest or getting a high yield. It is also about making the right decisions to produce the best food you can.

The soil, climate, sun, humidity, fertilizer, watering habits, and the selected cultivar are unique to your garden. For this reason it is difficult for anyone else to give you specific instructions for growing high quality food.

For example, I see discussions online about suckering tomatoes (the removal of side branches) and its effect of yield, fruit size, or harvest time. What is almost never discussed is the effect on the quality of the fruit. How does suckering affect nutrition? We really don't know.

I hope this discussion does not discourage you from growing your own food. I only want to make you aware of the fact that your decisions in the garden do affect food quality, but in many cases you will have a hard time knowing what the effect is. How do you resolve this issue? Do things in the garden that make plants grow to their full potential. Better growing plants generally produce food that is of a higher quality and more nutritious.

The History of Food Science

Food and nutrition has been studied for centuries, but modern food science is a very young science. It is one reason why we still know so little about it. The first vitamin was isolated and qualified one hundred years ago. This led to the study of nutrient deficiency for a handful of nutrients, mostly vitamins. The problem with this is that a healthy body is affected by thousands of compounds and they all have some role to play in our health. Studying a few nutrients is valuable, but does not come close to helping us understand the whole picture.

By the 1960s and 1970s, we understood the role of vitamins and started adding them as supplements to food. Malnutrition due to vitamin deficiency dropped dramatically in developed countries, but it is still a problem in a large part of the world.

Then scientists started focusing on the role of fat and sugar in our diet. Early studies showed that fat was a major contributor to heart disease. Sugar was implicated in coronary disease, cancer, and dental caries. Low fat, low cholesterol, low sugar diets became the standard while artificial sugars and margarine became staples.

This science seemed to flip-flop and soon fat was not so bad in our diet. Cholesterol became "good" cholesterol and "bad" cholesterol. And now, too much artificial sweetener and margarine are not good for you.

From the public's perspective, science got it wrong, and in some ways they did. The problem is that the science looked at one or two aspects of health and tried to make conclusions about the effect of thousands of compounds. Human bodies and health-related chemistries are extremely complex. Looking at one or two aspects makes it hard to reach any valid conclusion.

It is important to remember that many people were dying from health-related illnesses and we wanted to provide some kind of help. Even though the recommendations for fat and sugar were not perfect, they did save lives and they did advance science. That is one of the fundamental beauties of science—it is an iterative process that slowly fine-tunes our knowledge.

Today we know a lot more about nutrition, but we are still just starting to understand the complexities of food science. As you read through this book you will repeatedly find that our so-called understanding of food science is really just a glimmer of information. Today's emphatic statements of fact are really just guesses at the full truth. They are, however, the best we have today.

2
Understanding Nutrition

The National Institute of Health defines nutrition as "the field of study focusing on foods and substances in foods that help animals (and plants) to grow and stay healthy." Nutrition is the science that looks at the components of food and how they affect our bodies. It also defines the quality of food and determines which foods are better for us while at the same time identifying foods or components of food that are harmful to us.

We talk a lot about food, but it is important to understand that a food item is a collection of chemicals and each of these chemicals reacts differently in our bodies. Nutrition is really the study of chemicals found in food and their effect on our bodies.

To simplify discussions, nutritionists have categorized these chemicals into several main groups, including protein, carbohydrates, fiber, fats, minerals, vitamins, and water. Except for water, each group consists of many different compounds and each of these compounds is a nutrient for our bodies. For example, vitamin C is a nutrient in the vitamin group. Sucrose is a nutrient in the carbohydrate group.

These nutrients are not isolated compounds. Many react with each other, forming a complex system. Calcium is an interesting example in this regard. It is an important nutrient for us, but there is a difference between the amount in food and the amount that is available to us, something we call bioavailability.

In plants, calcium combines with other molecules such as phytate, fiber, proteins, fatty acids, and oxalate. You might recognize oxalate as oxalic acid, the toxic substance in rhubarb leaves. When calcium binds with oxalic acid to form calcium oxalate, the calcium is no longer bioavailable in our gut. Our bodies can't digest it. So even if a plant has high levels of calcium oxalate, our bodies get no nutritional value from it.

Phytate is an antioxidant molecule that is called an "antinutrient" because it binds with calcium and makes it biounavailable to us. Unrefined cereals and legumes contain the highest concentrations of phytate. Eating a lot of these foods will reduce the calcium you absorb during digestion.

When I was growing up spinach was called a "superfood" because it contained high amounts of iron, which is the nutrient that gave Popeye his super-human strength. It turns out that spinach does contain a fair amount of iron, but it is not super high. Iron is another nutrient that binds with oxalic acid, and our bodies can only absorb about 2 percent of the iron found in spinach.

Here are some things you can do to make food more bioavailable:

- chop or mince food that has a rigid structure like leaves and stems
- soak grains in water and discard the water (phytate is water-soluble)
- cook foods like beans to reduce polyphenols
- balance raw and cooked foods to maximize the absorption of micronutrients
- eat citrus foods high in vitamin C along with iron-containing foods

Human Nutrients vs Plant Nutrients

Gardeners routinely talk about plant nutrients, and these include things like nitrate, phosphate, iron, and zinc. These are all small molecules that are able to enter a plant through the root system. Plants are also able to absorb molecules that are slightly larger, including things such as glucose and amino acids.

What happens when a large protein nutrient is given to a plant? Nothing. Proteins are just too big to get through the wall of a root.

Plants have to wait until microbes break up the protein, first into amino acids and finally into small molecules such as nitrate and sulfur. It is only then that plants are able to use the protein as food. Because plants can't use proteins directly, proteins are not plant nutrients. Only nitrate is a plant nutrient.

Humans and other animals process food differently. We can take a big bite out of a chicken leg and chew it up along with saliva, which starts the digestion process. The stomach then adds digestive juices containing hydrochloric acid and the enzyme pepsin, which starts breaking down the protein. The protein molecule is slowly broken down into smaller and smaller pieces. The resulting mixture in the stomach is called chyme.

The digestion of protein in the stomach takes longer than the digestion of carbohydrates, but not as long as the digestion of fats. This explains why a high protein meal makes you feel full longer.

The chyme now passes into the small intestine where the majority of the protein will be digested. The pancreas secretes more enzymes (chymotrypsin and trypsin) into the mix to further break down the protein fragments. The lining of the small intestine adds even more enzymes that finally break the protein down into amino acids, which are then absorbed into the blood. Our bodies can use amino acids as building blocks to make new proteins.

When we are talking about animals, the term nutrient includes many larger molecules that the digestive system can absorb. In terms of human nutrition, all usable food molecules are nutrients.

Nutrients vs Calories

Nutrients are molecules the body needs to survive. Calories is a measure of the amount of energy stored in those molecules. Our bodies need energy to function, stay warm, and carry out all chemical reactions. If you need 2,400 calories a day, you can get this by eating a wide variety of food including candy, chicken, and vegetables. The right amount of each of these foods will give you the right amount of calories, but each food item supplies different types of nutrients.

Counting calories is not a good way to evaluate a diet. It is actually better to eat more calories of healthy food than fewer calories of less healthy food. Eating more calories than you need increases body weight. A gram of fat contains nearly twice as many calories as a gram of carbohydrate or protein.

Nutrients in Food

Proteins

Proteins are large complex molecules that do most of the work in cells. We know them under different names including enzymes, antibodies, transporters, and messengers. Antibodies bind to specific foreign particles such as viruses and bacteria, and protect us from them. Enzymes carry out most of the chemical reactions in a cell. Messenger proteins can function as hormones to coordinate biological functions, thereby controlling things such as growth. Structural proteins are key components of cell walls, and on a larger scale they provide structure to muscles. Transport proteins move specific molecules across cell membranes, allowing our digestive systems—and plant roots—to absorb nutrients.

Each type of protein is made up of a long chain of hundreds or thousands of amino acids. Once the chain is made, it folds up in a 3-D structure that is unique for each protein. That structure is critical in determining the functionality and properties of the protein. Proteins are made out of mostly carbon, hydrogen, nitrogen, oxygen, and sulfur. A few contain phosphorus, iron, copper, or zinc. They affect the flavor and texture of food, and sulfur and nitrogen are important nutrients.

The human body has about 100,000 different proteins, while our DNA codes for only 20,000 proteins. Our cells are able to take the DNA template for one protein and use it to make several different ones by cutting and splicing pieces together. The total number of protein molecules in a single cell is estimated at 42 million. Most exist as a few thousand molecules, but some are plentiful at more than half a million copies.

There are twenty different types of amino acids. Eleven of these are made in our body and the others, called "essential amino acids," must be obtained from our food. The nine essential amino acids are histidine, isoleucine, leucine, lysine, methionine, phenylalanine, threonine, tryptophan, and valine. Each protein contains a different amount of each amino acid, so the amount of each amino acid required in our diet is different. For example, the recommended daily amount for every 2.2 pounds of body weight is 42 mg for leucine and only 5 mg for tryptophan.

The three-dimensional structure of proteins is essential for them to carry out their function. The term denaturation is used for a process whereby proteins unfold, and this can be caused by pH, heat, freezing, physical agitation, and high salt concentrations. Heating egg whites denatures protein, producing white solids. Making cottage cheese by adding acid to milk is the result of a denatured protein. Beating the proteins in egg whites forms meringue. Once a protein is denatured, it will not reform properly and its original characteristics are lost.

Percent Protein in Various Foods[1]

Food type	Percent protein	Food type	Percent protein
Beans	7	Nuts	15
Broccoli	2	Pasta	5
Cheese	25	Peas	5
Eggs	14	Potato	3
Fish	24	Rice	11
Fruit	1	Spinach	3
Meat	30	Yogurt	5

Enzymes

All enzymes are proteins, but not all proteins are enzymes. Each enzyme is specific for a particular reaction, although what we think of as a single reaction might actually be a set of reactions. For example, photosynthesis is a complex process that requires several enzymes. The "oxygen evolving complex," consisting of several enzymes, breaks up water molecules to start the photosynthesis process. "ATP Synthase," another enzyme, converts ATP to ADP to release the energy needed for the reaction. "Rubisco" combines carbon from CO_2 to form sugar molecules.

Enzymes carry out reactions that affect molecular structure, flavor, taste, and texture. They can increase or decrease important nutrients, and they are reused over and over again. You can think of them as taxis moving molecules from place to place. It drives around until flagged down by someone. That passenger might go and pick up a second person and then both are dropped off at a new location for a date. The taxi is now free to do it all over again. A big difference between a taxi and enzymes is that enzymes are specific to a particular type of passenger (molecule).

Understanding enzymes can be important in cooking. For example, gelatin is a protein that absorbs water and other small molecules as it sets into a solid gel. Pineapple contains a protein-digesting enzyme called bromelain that reacts with proteins to break them up into small peptide molecules. What happens when you try to make a gelatin salad with pineapple? Bromelain reacts with gelatin and breaks it down so that it can no longer form a gel and your gelatin salad stays runny.

Canned pineapple doesn't have the same effect because heat from the canning process denatures (inactivates) bromelain. Canned pineapple works just fine in a gelatin salad, as does cooked pineapple. Other plants also produce similar enzymes called proteases that prevent gelatin from setting. These include fresh papaya, mango, guava, and kiwi.

Bromelain is also used as a meat tenderizer. In fact, some people are very sensitive to the enzyme and find that it makes their lips and tongue sore. This is because the bromelain is tenderizing your tongue! Why does it not also tenderize your stomach? The acids there denature it.

Complete Proteins

A food is considered to be a complete protein source when it contains all nine essential amino acids in amounts relative to what our bodies need. An incomplete protein source has some of these amino acids but not all of them. Meat, poultry, fish, eggs, and milk are complete protein sources and for this reason many people believe that we need to have some of these in our diet.

Most sources of plant protein are not complete:

- legumes are a good source of lysine, and a poor source of tryptophan and sulfur-containing amino acids.
- nuts and seeds contain tryptophan and sulfur-containing amino acids.
- cereals and grains are a good source of tryptophan and sulfur-containing amino acid, and a poor source of lysine.
- starchy vegetables have lower levels of lysine and methionine.
- green leafy vegetables contain tryptophan, leucine, threonine, and phenylalanine, but are low in the others.

There are some complete plant-based sources, including:

- quinoa
- buckwheat
- hempseed
- blue-green algae
- soybeans

A common belief is that every meal needs to include all of the essential amino acids so that they are consumed at the same time, but that is a myth. It's been shown that an optimal amino acid profile is perfectly obtainable by eating a variety of protein sources over the course of a day. A single serving of meat will provide all of the essential amino acids. Vegetarian or vegan diets should include a variety of different protein sources so that the total amount of amino acids consumed in a day meets the daily requirements.

Carbohydrates

Carbohydrates are organic compounds that contain carbon, oxygen, and hydrogen and include important food constituents such as sugars, dextrins, starches, celluloses, pectins, and gums. These provide both energy and fiber in our diets. Most of the dry weight of plants as well as the pages of this book are made up of carbohydrates.

Table sugar (sucrose) is called a disaccharide because it contains the two simple sugars: glucose and fructose. These three sugars are critical for all life forms, including bacteria, plants, and animals. They are broken down in a process called respiration to produce energy (4 calories/g) and carbon dioxide.

Sucrose (table sugar)

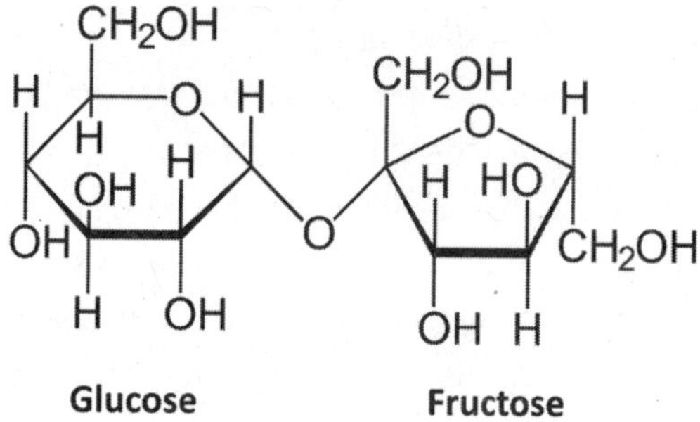

The molecular structure of sucrose (glucose + fructose)

Sugars are sweet, and fructose is the main sugar that gives fruits their sweet taste. In solution they are viscous and provide food with a desirable mouthfeel. Microbes can also use sugar as an energy source, but at high concentrations sugar prevents microbes from growing. That is why jams and jellies keep so well.

Sugar molecules can be joined together to form longer chains called polysaccharides. An example of this is raffinose that contains galactose, glucose, and fructose. It is found in dried beans and peas. Our bodies are unable to digest it, so it travels through the stomach into the large intestine where bacteria break it down, producing gas. You might be familiar with the jingle, "beans, beans, good for the heart. The more you eat the more you...." You get the picture.

Starches, pectins, and gums are more complicated polysaccharides that are found in all living things. There are hundreds of different types and when we eat them, enzymes break the long chains of molecules into smaller and smaller chains. We are then able to use these small molecules to build the new polysaccharides that we need. The take-home message here is that too much sugar is not good for us, but without a steady supply of these carbohydrates, we cannot live.

The term fiber is used for carbohydrates that travel through the digestive tract but are not digested or absorbed. They therefore don't provide energy or nutrients, but they are very important for making our digestive system work properly. Fiber provides bulk for muscles of the digestive tract to squeeze against, which helps move food through the system. They are found in roots, stems, leaves, nuts, and the outer seed covering of vegetables, fruits, and whole grains.

Fiber also acts like a sponge for unhealthy substances, reducing their absorption into our body. For example, fiber reduces the absorption of cholesterol into the bloodstream, lowering the chance of getting colon cancer.

Food Myth: Brown Sugar Is Healthier

Most table sugar is made from sugar cane and sugar beets. Both are ground up and a liquid is extracted and refined to form white sugar. During the refining process, a brown liquid waste product called molasses is also produced. Brown sugar is made by coating refined white sugar with varying amounts of molasses. The amount of molasses in brown sugar is very small and therefore does not provide much nutrition.

Molasses is 22 percent water, 75 percent sugar, and about 2 percent minerals, including selenium, calcium, magnesium, iron, manganese, potassium, and copper. Sulfur may be added to the molasses to help control bacteria growth during the manufacturing process.

Natural sugar is found in fruits and vegetables and is claimed to be healthier, but it is the exact same sugar, namely sucrose, found in refined white sugar. The fact that it comes from fruits and vegetables does not make it any healthier.

From a nutritional point of view, natural sugar, refined white sugar, and brown sugar are all the same sugar. None is more nutritious than the others.

Fats & Oils

Fats and oils are essentially the same thing and are collectively called triglycerides. Each triglyceride is made up of a molecule of glycerol and three fatty acids. They consist of carbon, hydrogen, and oxygen, which are the same components of carbohydrates. A triglyceride is called a fat if it is a solid at room temperature (77°F, 25°C) and an oil if it is a liquid at room temperature. Fats come from meat, lard, butter, coconut oil, and palm oil, while oils come from fish and plants.

You have probably heard terms like "saturated fats" or "unsaturated fatty acids." The term saturated refers to the amount of hydrogen atoms in the molecule. A higher number of hydrogen atoms results in a higher "degree of saturation." Saturated fatty acids have more hydrogen and tend to be found in saturated fats. Unsaturated fatty acids have fewer hydrogen atoms and are found in unsaturated fats, which tend to be called oils. In general, unsaturated fats are healthier. The degree of saturation has a significant effect on the properties of food such as flavor, mouthfeel, texture, and aroma. Higher fat levels make doughnuts taste better!

Humans are able to synthesize most of the fatty acids, but there are two that are essential in our diet. They include linoleic acid, an omega-6 fatty acid, and α-linolenic acid, an omega-3 fatty acid. The former is found in soybean oil, corn oil, and safflower oil, and the latter is found in soybean oil, canola oil, walnuts, and flaxseed. Note that meat is not a good source for either of these.

Fats are important in our diet because they provide fat-soluble vitamins and they are an important energy source. Fat has about 9 calories per gram while carbohydrates and protein have about 4 calories per gram. Fat is an important part of cell membranes and is found in high concentrations in brain and nerve tissue. Excess fat is stored in our bodies and too much has a negative health effect.

Fruits and vegetables are a better source of unsaturated triglycerides, but vegetables only contain about 5% fat (dry weight) and fruits are even less at 1%.

Vitamins

Vitamins are organic substances that our bodies need in small amounts. They are essential in our diet because we are either unable to synthesize them or we can't make enough to meet our needs. The list of vitamins is unique to each organism. For example, humans need to get vitamin C from their diets while dogs can produce their own vitamin C.

In some cases we don't need the vitamin in our diet because we can use other similar molecules to make the vitamin. The term used for these other molecules is provitamin or previtamin. For example, beta-carotene is a provitamin A. Our bodies have an enzyme that can convert beta-carotene into vitamin A. Most discussions do not distinguish between a vitamin and a provitamin. The term vitamin A is used for both beta-carotene and vitamin A.

Vitamins are classified as either fat soluble or water soluble. Fat-soluble vitamins (A, D, E, K) dissolve in fat and tend to accumulate in the body. They are more abundant in food that contains fat. Water-soluble vitamins, including C and the B-complex, dissolve in water. They are not stored, and any unused amounts are expelled in the urine. We therefore require a daily dose of these vitamins.

This difference in solubility is important in preserving food. Soaking or boiling food in water tends to remove the water-soluble vitamins more than the fat-soluble ones. Vitamins are also degraded by enzymes. Blanching food prior to freezing destroys enzymes and helps preserve vitamins.

Many people in developed countries take daily vitamin supplements because it's become fashionable, but in most cases they are unnecessary. A good healthy diet provides all the vitamins your body can use. If you are not getting enough vitamins you will get sick. On the other hand, you can also get sick by eating too much of some vitamins. Since fat-soluble vitamins are stored, they can accumulate to toxic levels.

Some of the food available in grocery stores has been fortified with vitamins. This means that the manufacturer has added additional vitamins to the product. Milk usually contains added vitamin D, and bread is fortified with B9.

Vitamin A, also called retinol, is essential for growth and development, healthy vision, immune function, healthy teeth and bones, and reproduction. It helps the heart, lungs, and kidneys function properly. A deficiency of vitamin A causes eye problems and can lead to night blindness. Cataracts are responsible for 50 percent of blindness cases, and vitamin A and C can help prevent them.

Vitamin A is only available from animal sources, and the best sources include organ meats (liver), fatty fish (tuna), milk, cheese, and eggs. Humans are able to make vitamin A from beta-carotene and alpha-carotene, which are collectively known as provitamin A. These are the orange pigments found in carrots, oranges, squash, and red peppers. Provitamin A is also found in mango, broccoli, and spinach.

Vitamin C (ascorbic acid) helps your body fight infection and prevents diseases such as scurvy. It contributes to collagen production (muscles), helps wounds heal, strengthens blood vessels, and helps bone formation. It is important for iron absorption and acts as an antioxidant. Scurvy results in bleeding gums, loss of teeth, and wounds that don't heal. This used to be a common disease with sailors two hundred years ago until the British discovered that citrus fruits prevented it.

Fruits and vegetables are good sources of vitamin C with citrus and berries having the highest level. Cooking destroys it.

The idea of taking a daily dose of vitamin C to ward off a cold is a myth. It might shorten the time you are sick by a small amount, but a cold is an infection and no amount of vitamin C will prevent it. Most people in developed countries get enough vitamin C from the food they eat. The body can't store it, and any excess is expelled through urine.

Vitamin D (cholecalciferol) indirectly helps bones and teeth develop properly by helping intestines absorb calcium and phosphorus into the bloodstream. Human bodies can produce vitamin D, but they are not very efficient at doing so unless skin is exposed to UVB rays from the sun or other source. That can be a problem in cold climates in winter, but even exposing the face to one hour of sunlight is enough to produce the daily requirement of vitamin D.

A vitamin D deficiency can cause rickets and osteomalacia, a softening of the bones. A good source for vitamin D includes fatty fish (salmon, tuna), egg yolks, cheese, beef liver, and mushrooms. Processed foods may be fortified with vitamin D.

Vitamin E (tocopherol) scavenges free radicals (loose electrons) that can damage cells. By doing so it enhances the immune system, prevents clots, decreases inflammation, and may prevent diseases.

Vitamin E is mainly stored in the liver until it is released into the bloodstream. Deficiencies are rare, but they can cause muscle weakness, problems with coordination, and numbness. Vitamin E is found in plant-based oils, nuts, seeds, wheat germ, fruits, and vegetables.

Vitamin K comes in two types. Phylloquinone is found in green leafy vegetables such as collard greens, kale, and spinach, and in oils such as soybean and canola, while menaquinone is found in meat, cheese, eggs, and fermented foods. Vitamin K is important for developing proteins that are used for blood clotting and bone development. It is found throughout the body, including the liver, brain, heart, pancreas, and bones. Excess vitamin K is quickly broken down and excreted in urine and stool.

An important source for this vitamin are the bacteria in our gut. Antibiotics can destroy the bacteria, resulting in deficiencies, especially if the drug is taken for more than a couple of weeks. Since vitamin K is fat-soluble, it is a good idea to consume some fat or oil with meals to help absorb it.

B vitamins include B1 (thiamin), B2 (riboflavin), B3 (niacin), B5 (pantothenic acid), B6 (pyridoxine), B7 (biotin), B9 (folate, folic acid), B12 (cobalamin). These vitamins help a variety of enzymes complete their task, ranging from releasing energy to breaking down amino acids and transporting oxygen around the body. Some of these may also play a role in reducing cancer and heart disease.

The B vitamins are found in a wide variety of foods, both animal and plant based, so the best approach is to eat a varied diet. They are also added as supplements to many processed foods. A deficiency can have a variety of symptoms, including skin rashes, scaly skin on lips, weakness, confusion, depression, nausea, and numbness of hands and feet.

Folate is a natural B vitamin found in many foods. Unfortunately, our digestive system is not efficient at absorbing it and we don't store it for long. A manufactured form of this vitamin called folic acid is used to fortify foods and it has the advantage that our bodies are better at absorbing it. This is a good example of a manufactured chemical that is better than the natural form.

Important Mineral Nutrients for Humans[2]

Mineral	What it does	Where it's found
Macrominerals		
Sodium	controls fluid balance, nerve transmission, muscle contraction	table salt, processed foods, bread, vegetables, unprocessed meats
Calcium	part of bones and teeth, muscle contraction, nerve function, blood clotting, blood pressure	milk products, greens, legumes
Chlorine	proper fluid balance, stomach acid	table salt, processed foods, bread, vegetables, unprocessed meats
Magnesium	important in bones, making proteins, nerve transmission, immune system	nuts, seeds, legumes, leafy vegetables, seafood, hard water
Phosphorus	teeth and bones, acid-base balance, DNA, ATP (our energy source)	meats, fish, poultry, eggs, milk
Potassium	fluid balance, nerve transmission, muscle contraction	meats, milk, fresh fruits and vegetables, whole grains, legumes
Sulfur	found in proteins	meats, poultry, fish, eggs, milk, legumes and nuts
Microminerals		
Iron	hemoglobin found in red blood cells, movement of oxygen, energy metabolism	meats, fish, poultry, shellfish, egg yolks, legumes, dried fruits, dark leafy greens, iron-enriched breads, cereals
Zinc	part of many enzymes, taste perception, wound healing, normal fetal development, production of sperm, normal growth and sexual maturation, immune system health	meats, fish, poultry, leavened whole grains, vegetables
Chromium	works with insulin to regulate blood sugar	liver, brewer's yeast, whole grains, nuts, cheese
Copper	part of many enzymes, iron metabolism	legumes, nuts, seeds, whole grains, organ meats, drinking water
Fluoride	formation of bones and teeth, helps prevent tooth decay	drinking water, fish, most teas
Iodine	thyroid hormone, regulate growth, development, and metabolism	seafood, foods grown in iodine-rich soil, iodized salt, bread, dairy products
Manganese	part of many enzymes	most food, especially plant-based food
Molybdenum	part of enzymes	legumes, bread, grains, leafy green vegetables, milk, liver
Selenium	an antioxidant	meats, seafood, grains

Minerals

Minerals are inorganic elements that are mostly the same as the nutrients used by plants, including calcium, magnesium, potassium, phosphorus, etc. Plants absorb these from the soil and they are in turn eaten by animals. Fruits, vegetables, and meats provide the minerals in our diet. Just like plants, we need some of these minerals in larger amounts and call them macrominerals, and those needed in smaller amounts are called microminerals.

Minerals play many important roles. Sodium and potassium carry charges that make nerves and muscles work. Iron is part of the hemoglobin molecule that carries oxygen in red blood cells. Calcium and phosphorus along with vitamin D are critical for building strong bones and teeth. Several minerals are part of enzymes that carry out a wide range of reactions.

The body usually recycles minerals. For example, when red blood cells are about four months old, they are broken down. Iron is extracted and blood transports it to bone marrow where it is recycled into new hemoglobin molecules.

Minerals can also be tied up by other molecules that we eat. You might know that vegetables such as spinach and rhubarb contain oxalic acid. Seeds, nuts, legumes, and unprocessed bran contain a chemical called phytic acid. Both of these compounds bind with calcium in our gut, preventing its absorption.

Phytonutrients

Many of the compounds that have been discussed so far are essential in our diets, but there are many other compounds in our diet that are beneficial but not essential. One group of these are called phytonutrients or phytochemicals. "Phyto" refers to the Greek word for plant. Most of these chemicals are produced naturally by the plant to ward off pests and diseases, but in our diet they can be very beneficial to our health and help us fight off certain diseases.

We have now identified more than twenty-five thousand phytonutrients, and to be honest we don't know what most of them do. The science on these compounds is just starting to emerge.

Many claims have been made for these compounds. Some seem to help cancer cells self-destruct. Others react with carcinogens before they can affect cells. They may even block the formation of tumors in blood vessels. Notice that I used the words "seem to" and "may." We have to be very careful about these claims because most of this is very preliminary science.

Quite a few phytochemicals have been shown to work well in the lab, only to find out that they are not even absorbed by the gut. In other cases, helpful bacteria in our gut break them down before they can be absorbed and provide a benefit to us. The side effects of these compounds have not been studied well at all. We still have a lot to learn about this group of compounds, but the general sense is that they are valuable in our diet and the best way to get a lot of different ones is to eat a varied diet.

To help quantify the benefits of such a large number of compounds, scientists have developed the Phytochemical Index (PI), which is defined as the percent of dietary calories derived from foods rich in phytochemicals. These foods include fruits, most vegetables, fruit/vegetable juices, legumes, whole grains, nuts, seeds, soy products, wine, beer, and cider. It excludes refined oils, sugars, grains, potato products, hard liquors, and animal products. There are some apps that let you input your food intake and then calculate the PI.

This is a list of some of the more common groups of phytonutrients:

- carotenoid pigments
- flavonoid pigments
- sulforaphane
- isothiocyanates in the cabbage family
- saponins in legumes
- limonene and phenols in citrus

"Eating the rainbow" has become a popular expression. The idea is that you should eat a lot of different colored fruits and vegetables. This does not include colorful jujubes! Many of the phytonutrients are compounds that have a color, and if you eat the rainbow you are eating a lot of different healthy nutrients.

Colorful food is good for us, but so are white vegetables. Cauliflower, mushrooms, and garlic also have nutritional benefits, including fiber, potassium, and magnesium.

Antioxidants

What are antioxidants? The term has become popular and is associated with nutrition and health, but few actually understand what they are. In simple terms, antioxidants are compounds that neutralize free radicals.

Free radicals are compounds that travel through your body, trying to strip electrons from other compounds. When they are successful, many of these other compounds become harmful to our bodies and cause a variety of chronic diseases. Free radicals can change DNA, cause LDL (the bad cholesterol) to stick to artery walls, and they can alter cell membranes, which changes the movement of molecules into and out of cells.

Our bodies produce antioxidants to keep the quantity of free radicals in check so that they don't do too much harm. We can also get antioxidants from food since every other living organisms is also producing them to control their own free radicals.

It is important to understand that there are many different kinds of free radicals and many different kinds of antioxidants. Free radicals are only neutralized when a matching type of antioxidant is present. What this means is that increasing the wrong antioxidant in your diet won't be of any help. What you really need is lots of different ones so that the right one is available when needed.

There are hundreds if not thousands of different antioxidants. Some familiar ones include vitamin C, vitamin E, beta-carotene, selenium, manganese, flavonoids, phenols, and many more.

Some foods have higher amounts of antioxidants and they have been labeled as "superfoods," including things like cocoa, berries, spices, and legumes. Along with that title came all kinds of health claims and people started promoting higher consumption of superfoods. Blueberries topped the list and were heavily promoted as disease-fighters. The reality is that the science supporting these claims is very weak or nonexistent.

It is clear that excessive free radicals contribute to chronic diseases, including cancer, heart disease, cognitive decline, and vision loss and that natural antioxidants in our bodies help reduce diseases. However, there is little scientific support for the idea that eating more antioxidants or using supplements containing antioxidants will reduce diseases.[3]

Water

You might be surprised that I have included water here, but it is essential for life. Plants are 80–90 percent water, while seeds only have about 10 percent. Our bodies contain about 60 percent water, with the brain and heart having 73 percent, the lungs 83 percent, the skin 64 percent, and bones 31 percent. For comparison, fish are about 78 percent water, which is less than plants.

Water is needed for digestion, carrying waste, making urine, circulating blood, controlling body temperature, and for controlling many chemical reactions taking place in cells. If you lose too much water, cells shrink and may no longer function properly. Keep in mind that we get water from both drinking and eating. All of our food contains some water, and we get about 20 percent of our water from food (such as soup).

Moisture content is also important if you are looking at the cost of food. Which is cheaper: lettuce, apples, or peanuts? The price of nuts has skyrocketed, so they must be more expensive, right? Not really. Water is cheap, so we need to remove it from the food before we compare prices. The table below shows that peanuts are actually cheaper on a dry weight basis. Lettuce is extremely high in cost.

The Real Cost of Food

Food	Cost/500 g	Moisture content	Cost/100g dry weight
Washed, cut iceberg lettuce	$3.00	95%	$12.00
Shelled peanuts	$3.00	10%	$0.66
Honeycrisp apples	$2.00	80%	$2.00

Note: The above prices are from Walmart, in US dollars.

Food Myth: You Should Drink 8 Glasses of Water a Day

Our bodies lose about half a gallon (2 litres) of water per day, mostly through sweating, breathing, and urination. This is higher in hot climates, with extra exercise, and with a fever. This water needs to be replenished, and about 20 percent comes from solid food. Normal consumption of juice, milk, tea, or coffee provides the rest of the requirement. Even the original recommendation of drinking eight glasses a day (1945, US Food and Nutrition Board) stated that most of our water intake could come from food sources.

You do not need to drink eight glasses of water each day. Here are some other myths about drinking water:

- Being thirsty does not mean you are dehydrated. Spicy and salty foods will make you thirsty. If you are thirsty, drink some water but don't worry about being dehydrated.
- You can drink too much water, which leads to hyponatremia where salt levels are too low. At high doses, water is toxic and can kill you.
- Coffee and other caffeinated beverages consumed in moderation provide the same hydration as noncaffeinated drinks. They do not dehydrate you.
- Many people now drag a water bottle along wherever they go because "you need to drink every few minutes." This is a complete myth even during normal exercise.
- Tap water in developed countries is highly regulated and is usually just as good if not better than bottled water. Years ago I saw a chemical analysis of Toronto, Ontario, drinking water compared to bottled water. Although both are safe to drink, the bottled water contained higher levels of toxins, many coming from the plastic in the bottle. Bottled water also costs a lot more.

Factors Affecting Nutrients

Many factors affect the nutrient level in food, starting with the selection of seed, the growing methods, harvesting, storage, and finally the cooking methods used to prepare the food. Food science studies the impact of all of these factors.

Food Myth: Brown Eggs Are More Nutritious

Chicken eggs are available in two common colors: brown and white. Some parts of the country prefer brown eggs because they are reported to be more nutritious. Other regions prefer white eggs. What is the difference?

Shell color depends on the breed of chicken. Brown-eared hens produce brown-shelled eggs. White eggs come from hens with white ears. Yes, chickens have ears; they are hidden under the feathers. There are also bluish eggs and matching colored hens. All of these eggs have the same flavor, quality, and nutrition provided they were raised the same way.

The color and nutrition of the yolk is affected by the feed given to the birds. A deep yellow pigment is due to beta-carotene, xanthophyll, or lycopene, three phytonutrients.

It all starts with the selection of seeds. Not only do you have to decide which food to grow, but you also need to select the cultivar (the variety). Each type of tomato will produce fruit that has different nutrient levels. For example, some tomatoes have a higher sugar level than others and they may taste sweeter. Each type of potato has different levels of solanine, a toxic compound I'll discuss later in the book.

Unfortunately for the gardener, there is very little information about the nutritional qualities of different cultivars. You can find the nutrient levels in peas online, but you are unlikely to find any useful information that compares the nutrient levels between snap peas and snow peas, let alone between Early Frosty and Green Arrow.

Once you have something growing, the next big impact on nutrition is climate and soil. Most of the nutrients in plants are compounds produced by the plant, and the production of these is very dependent on where the plant is grown. You have probably heard about low acid tomatoes, which is mostly a myth, but in the US you can find low acid tomatoes growing in a few locations. Grow the exact same cultivar in any other location and it won't have low acidity.

You have limited control over climate, but you can control the amount of water your plants get, and this can be important for nutrient levels. You also have limited control over soil, but again, you can improve the quality of your soil to grow more nutritious food. I won't discuss the topic of soil very much since it is fully covered in my other book, *Soil Science for Gardeners*.

Harvesting fruits and vegetables at the right time can have a big impact on nutrition. It is also very important to either eat the food right away, or to process and store it correctly to maintain a high level of nutrition. Each of these topics has their own chapter in this book.

Nutrition Myths

Myth #1: Avoid Total Fat and Saturated Fat

Fat provides energy and fat-soluble vitamins. In moderation it is good for you.

Myth #2: Eggs Raise Cholesterol Level

Eggs are high in cholesterol, but eating them does not seem to raise cholesterol levels. They are also full of minerals, vitamins, and antioxidants.

Myth #3: Lose Weight by Eating Less Fat

The cry for using low fat diets to lose weight has backfired. Companies replace fat with carbohydrates such as sugar to replace the good taste of fats. Overeating these "better for you" foods has actually led to more obesity.

Fat from foods such as nuts, vegetable oil, and fish are essential in the diet. Fat also helps you feel full longer, which reduces snacking.

Myth #4: Only People with High Blood Pressure Should Limit Their Sodium

Many healthy people consume more sodium than recommended and it can lead to future stroke, heart disease, and kidney disease. Most of the sodium we eat comes from processed food, but even fresh fruits and vegetables contain some sodium.

Myth #5: Honey Is Better than White Sugar

Table sugar is sucrose, a type of sugar. Most of the sugar in honey, maple syrup, and coconut sugar is also sucrose. Honey does contain twenty-two amino acids, thirty-one different minerals and a wide range of vitamins and enzymes. However, these nutrients are only present in trace amounts and add no real nutritional value. None of these sources are much better than white sugar.

Myth #6: A Detox Diet Will Clean Toxins Out of the Body

The idea of removing toxins by eating special foods has no scientific support. Your existing liver, kidneys, and gastrointestinal tract do a good job of removing toxins without any special help from you.

Myth #7: Red Meat Is Harmful

The right kind of meat in moderation is not harmful. Fresh red meat, steak, and hamburger, do not cause heart disease, but processed meat can. The salts and nitrates in processed meat such as bacon, salami, and lunch meats are related to higher heart disease. A few small servings of these a week are fine, but it is better to reduce these in the diet and to limit the overall amount of meat you eat.

Myth #8: Fresh Fruits and Vegetables Are Always Healthier

This is a very common belief, but studies have shown that canned, frozen, or dried food can be just as nutritious. Preserving these foods properly is important, and I'll discuss details about that in other parts of the book.

Myth #9: Potato Skins Are Much More Nutritious than the Flesh

The skin does have higher levels of fiber, but most of the other nutrients including potassium and vitamin C are found in the flesh. It might also surprise you that a potato has more potassium than a banana and more vitamin C than an orange.

3

Food Safety—Chemicals

The term food safety is an umbrella term that encompasses a number of different aspects such as microbe contamination, chemical poisons, heavy metals, and even microplastics. This chapter will deal with each of these except for contamination from microbes, which will be discussed in the next chapter.

The general public has a skewed fear of chemicals. They differentiate between manufactured and natural chemicals, and the former group is considered dangerous while the latter is perfectly safe. It is common to see gardeners spread chemicals from their kitchen all over the garden without any concern, but mention a synthetic chemical and it's rejected immediately as a toxic substance. I hear this phrase a lot: "I garden without chemicals." That is simply not true; the soil, fertilizer, compost, the plants, and even the water are all chemicals. Too much water will kill you.

Pyrethrin is a natural pesticide that was originally made from chrysanthemums. Vinegar is a common spray used to kill weeds, although it does not work except on seedlings. Both pyrethrin and vinegar are more toxic than glyphosate, the active ingredient in Roundup. The seed from castor beans contains a chemical called ricin, which is one of the most deadly chemicals we know. Nicotine is just one of thousands of chemicals found in the tobacco plant. In the low doses found in cigarette smoke, it does very little harm short term, but long term it causes cancer. Ingesting 100 mg of pure nicotine will kill an adult almost instantly.

Not all natural chemicals are safe, and not all synthetic chemicals are harmful. The multivitamin you take each day is mostly synthetic chemicals. What is important is that you evaluate each chemical on its own merits—both synthetic and natural. We have to understand the value of the chemical as well as its potential harmful effects. Only then can we make a rational decision about how it should or should not be used.

The reality is that humans are exposed to thousands of chemicals at low doses every day. When you breathe the fresh air in your garden you inhale chemicals, both natural and manufactured. When you touch anything—plants, flowers, soil, mulch—you get chemicals on your skin and some of these will be absorbed through the skin. Everything you eat adds chemicals into your body, and many of the chemicals you eat are harmful. Both a banana and a tomato contain numerous toxic substances.

You are probably asking yourself, how can a banana be toxic and healthy at the same time? Toxicity depends very much on dose. In small amounts, many toxic chemicals will not harm us. In larger amounts they will. *The dose makes the poison.*

Tomatoes belongs to the deadly nightshade family, which includes a number of very poisonous plants (deadly nightshade, mandrake, henbane, datura), but also a number of edible plants such as: bell peppers (paprika), pointed peppers (spicy and sweet paprika), eggplant, and potatoes. All of these plants contain a substance called solanine, which is a natural pesticide produced by plants. There are many claims that if you eat enough green tomatoes it will poison you, causing unpleasant symptoms such as fever, abdominal pain, diarrhea, vomiting, drowsiness, and lethargy. The reality is that there is very little evidence of poisoning from green tomatoes. Most of the solanine passes through your gut without being absorbed.

Nightshade plants also contain nicotine, which also kills insects. That's right; when you eat a tomato, you eat some nicotine.

Tomatoes are rich in another alkaloid called tomatine. Green tomatoes contain quite a bit (500 mg/kg fresh fruit weight) to keep bugs from eating the fruit containing unripe seeds, but as the fruit matures the amount drops (5 mg/kg) because now the plant wants to encourage animals to distribute the seed. Ripe tomatoes have almost no tomatine.

Potatoes contain even more solanine than tomatoes and they also cause more fear of toxic poisoning. The reality is that an adult male would have to eat about sixty-seven large potatoes to be poisoned. There hasn't been a single case of solanine poisoning in the US from eating potatoes in the last fifty years.

The story about solanine and green tomatoes illustrates the fact that we should not fear chemicals. It is, however, important to understand them and their effect on both us and the environment.

Chemical Toxicity

There is a tendency to think of chemicals as either poisonous or harmless, but this is not correct because it implies an all or nothing effect. Any chemical can cause poisoning if the dose is high enough.

Sodium fluoride is a good example of this. At the very low doses found in toothpaste and drinking water, it causes no ill health effects. Quite the opposite; it provides a health benefit by strengthening our teeth, although that benefit is exaggerated. At higher repeated doses, fluoride builds up in our bones causing bone diseases.

Chemicals harm us in two general ways: short term and long term. We generally use the term poisoning for short-term effects. If you ingest cyanide, you die quickly and we call that a poisoning. If you are exposed to asbestos and it takes years to develop asbestosis, which eventually causes death, we call that a disease. Scientists use the terms acute toxicity and chronic toxicity.

Acute toxicity refers to a one-time exposure that can be through skin or eye contact or through ingestion. The effects are evident quickly. Acute toxicity is measured by exposing different animals (rats, fish, bees) to the chemical at different doses. This is referred to as the LD50. The LD50 is the dose at which half of the test animals die (lethal dose + 50%).

The LD50 is a convenient way to compare the toxicity of various chemicals. For example, the oral LD50 (rat) for cyanide is 56 mg/kg of body weight. Note that the value is given in terms of body weight since it takes less cyanide to kill a small rat than a large one. Vitamin C has an oral LD50 of 11,900 mg/kg. The number is higher for vitamin C, but this means it is less toxic. It takes more vitamin C to kill a rat than cyanide.

Gardeners love to use vinegar to try to kill weeds, but many would never use Roundup. How do these two chemicals compare as far as toxicity? Acetic acid, the active ingredient in vinegar, has an oral LD50 of 3,310 mg/kg. The oral LD50 of glyphosate, the active ingredient in Roundup, is 5,600 mg/kg. Vinegar is more toxic than glyphosate. That may surprise you, but these numbers are quite well established.

LD50 is a simple and effective way to compare the acute toxicity of chemicals. It does not consider the long-term effects of exposure to a chemical, which is chronic toxicity. Chronic toxicity is harder to measure since it happens very slowly over time. It is generally assessed by looking at populations of people and comparing their health conditions. For example, when you compare workers in the asbestos industry to workers in other fields, you find a higher incidence of asbestosis in people who have been exposed to asbestos. This indicates that asbestos causes long-term illnesses.

LD50 values are readily available online, but a good source for them is the National Pesticide Information Center.[1]

Government agencies such as the CDC and EPA examine chemicals and establish a "safe limit" for exposure that won't cause any harm, both short term and long term. They then lower this value by several magnitudes to add in a safety margin to make sure the value is safe. That gives them the published "safe level."

Chemicals Detected Everywhere

News outlets love to sensationalize the facts. They regularly report that a chemical has been found in drinking water, in food, and even in mother's milk. This makes for great headlines, but unfortunately it scares the general public and gives them a false understanding of the risks.

It is important to understand that our testing methods are now so good that we can detect almost every chemical, everywhere. Detection limits are down in the ppb level, which is equivalent to finding the right eight people among Earth's population. The fact that trace amounts of a chemical are found is quite meaningless unless you look at the dose.

A few years ago, drinking water sources in Spain were tested for glyphosate and it was found in most samples. News outlets had a field day with this fact and reported on how polluted drinking water was. I decided to write an article about this on my blog GardenMyths.com. I looked at the actual amount found and compared it to the safe limits established for the chemical. Then I calculated the amount of water you would need to drink to reach the "safe level." It turns out that you need to drink the equivalent of 1,000,000,000 12-ounce (355 ml) bottles every day just to get to the safe limit. Remember that this limit is orders of magnitude above the amount that would actually harm you. This is a nonissue that was exploited by news.

How Dirty Is the Dirty Dozen?

The "Dirty Dozen" is a list of the twelve most contaminated fruits and vegetables as determined by a special interest group called the Environmental Working Group (EWG). The list is released every year and they do an excellent job of scaring people into worrying about pesticides. Let's have a look at their logic and analysis.

Apples are usually at or near the top of the list. They claim that "97 percent of the apples sampled were found to contain pesticide residues." This testing is done by the United States Department of Agriculture, who runs a "Pesticide Data Program" and publishes the results.

In 2016, 531 apple samples were analyzed and none had a pesticide residue above the EPA's tolerance level. The tolerance level is the safe level for apples and it has a 100-fold safety margin built in.

A compound called diphenylamine was detected in 80 percent of samples. The EPA's tolerance level is 10 ppm, and the average detected value was 0.28 ppm. This means that there is no risk and yet the EWG found the apple to be one of the "most toxic" fruits and vegetables! Forbes had this to say: "The EWG analysis is egregiously misleading because it essentially counts all detections equally, ignoring what chemical it is, at what level it was detected, and how that compares to the crop-chemical-specific EPA tolerances."

The bottom line—the items on the Dirty Dozen list are not only safe to eat, but they don't even have to be washed to remove pesticides.

Pesticides

The general population fears pesticides in our food. It is true that historically we have used pesticides that were more toxic than we first thought. DDT is a good example of this. It was first used in the 1940s and was very effective at killing insects. It has an oral LD50 of about 500 mg/kg, which is "slightly to moderately" acutely toxic. The problem with DDT is that it persists in the environment and accumulates in fatty tissue. Over time it can cause tumors, and it is now classified as a probable human carcinogen. It did take scientists a while to figure this out.

This was followed by some organophosphate insecticides that were quite toxic. Most of these are no longer available. The newer class of pesticides are much safer and have undergone much more intensive testing, but many still feel uncomfortable about their use.

The idea that all pesticides are harmful is completely wrong. Many of today's pesticides have a short half-life, which means they don't last long in the environment. The dose on fruits and vegetables is extremely small. Many are easily digested in our bodies, or they may not even be absorbed and pass right through us.

Natural Pesticides

How do plants protect themselves from pests? They make natural pesticides. In fact, plants are fantastic chemical factories that make all kinds of nasty chemicals that kill insects and microbes. Remember that when they are attacked, plants can't run away. Their only defense is chemical warfare. You are probably familiar with the milkweed that contains a toxic latex-like compound that keeps almost everything from eating it. The exception is the monarch butterfly, which has developed the ability to tolerate it.

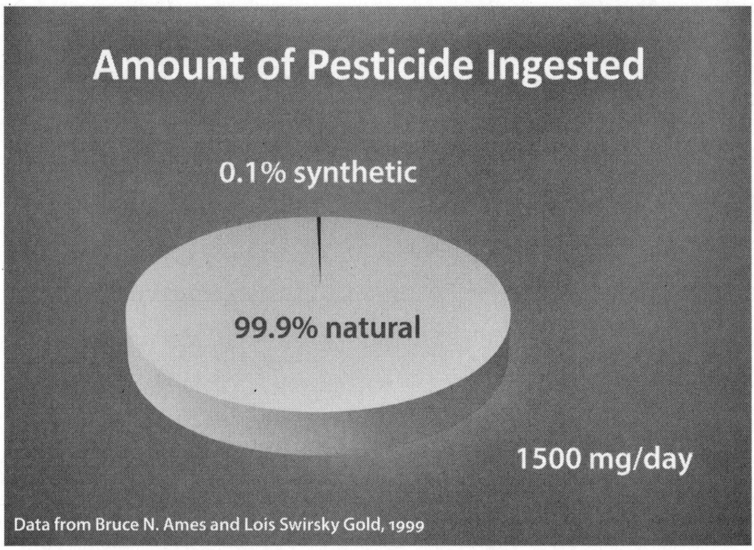

Amount of natural and synthetic pesticide ingested per day

There are thousands of these chemicals in every plant and each time we eat any part of a plant, we ingest these pesticides. On average we eat between five thousand and ten thousand different natural pesticides, most of which have not been adequately studied by science, so we don't know how dangerous they are. What we do know is that humans have been eating them for generations without significant problems. Please don't get alarmed by these numbers.

When we compare the amount of synthetic pesticides we ingest to the amount of natural pesticides, we find that the synthetic ones make up less than 0.1%. Society has been falsely conditioned to worry about this minor component of the pesticides we consume. Don't get me wrong, we need to be careful with synthetic pesticides and use them as little as possible, but they are not as significant in our diet as you've been led to believe.

You might be thinking that natural is better and safer, but this is another common myth. It is known as the "naturalistic fallacy." Many of these natural pesticides are carcinogens and some of the most toxic chemicals on the planet are natural compounds produced by plants. Take ricin for example. It is found in the beans of the castor bean, a common garden plant, and it is one of the most toxic chemicals on Earth.

Food Myth: Organic Food Does Not Have Pesticides

One of the main reasons people choose organic certified food is to eliminate the chemical pesticides on their food, thinking that organic food is not grown with chemical pesticides. That is not correct. Organic food can be grown with organically approved chemicals. Organic certified pesticides tend to be less effective than modern synthetic ones and are therefore used in higher doses.

Some of these chemicals are quite toxic. For example, copper sulfate has an oral LD50 of about 650 mg/kg, around the same as DDT. Copper is also a heavy metal, which is discussed below.

Organic food is safe to eat, but it is incorrect to think that it is grown without chemical pesticides.

Home Remedies

Many gardeners think that any home remedy is both safe and effective. Many are not. Just because chemicals came from the kitchen does not make it safe for use in the garden. Dish soap should not be eaten, although it is sprayed in vegetable gardens. Table salt is quite toxic to plants and soil life, and should not be spread around the garden. Mothballs are very toxic.

A larger concern is that more than 80 percent of home remedies do not even work. They are both a waste of time and resources. Just because someone on the internet or social media says it works does not mean it actually works. Gardeners rarely use controls and they almost never use enough plants to establish a significant result. Without those, the stated results are meaningless. If someone posts a remedy on the internet, ask them to describe the controls they used. If they can't explain the controls or didn't use them, don't believe them. For more on using controls see *The Scientific Method and Why Controls Are So Important.*[2]

Heavy Metals

The term heavy metal is not well defined, and different authors and professions use slightly different definitions. One chemical definition says heavy metals are elements having an atomic number greater than 20, have an atomic density above 5 g/cm^3, and have metallic properties. This would include copper, iron, manganese, cobalt, zinc, nickel, cadmium, lead, mercury, chromium, arsenic, and aluminum. Some people use the term for only the more toxic of these which includes arsenic, lead, mercury, and cadmium.

As a gardener you probably recognize some of these as plant nutrients: copper, iron, manganese, zinc, and aluminum. As with any chemical, dose makes the poison. These metals are required by plants in small amounts, but high doses are toxic. Aluminum sulfate is routinely recommended for acidifying soil and turning hydrangea flowers blue, but I would never add extra aluminum to my soil.

Unlike organic molecules, heavy metals are elements, and elements can't be decomposed, so they tend to accumulate in the environment. You might be familiar with the fact that mercury accumulates in fish. This starts with pollution on land. Industrial processes use mercury and some of it spills into the environment, eventually ending up in rivers and lakes. Small microbes ingest it, and it starts making its way up the food chain until it reaches fish. Since fish live a relatively long life, the mercury level in them keeps increasing until the fish are so toxic that we can't even eat them. This was a huge problem in the Great Lakes during the seventies and eighties. Levels are now much lower due to tighter pollution controls.

Chromium and arsenic are quite toxic to almost all life forms, including microbes. Prior to 2000, pressure-treated wood was made with compounds containing both of these heavy metals. They worked great in stopping wood rot. Unfortunately, they also leach chromium and lead into the surrounding soil. Around 2004, the industry switched to copper-based compounds that are almost as effective in stopping wood rot, but more importantly, they leach less, and copper is not nearly as toxic. Today's pressure-treated wood is considered safe to use for raised vegetable gardens.

Heavy metals are naturally ubiquitous in the environment and exist in soil, water, and air. They are also a common industrial pollutant. Plants absorb these heavy metals, and they end up in all of the fruits and vegetables you and farm animals eat. They then accumulate in our bodies. This is the reason for the great concern over heavy metals. The amount in a single apple is insignificant, but over a lifetime, the level of heavy metals in our body continues to increase. Arsenic, cadmium, chromium, and nickel are classified as group 1 carcinogens.

Another source of heavy metals are commercial products. Pesticides that were used in the eighties contained heavy metals since they are toxic to pests. Almost all of those products are now banned, but the residual heavy metal atoms are still in the soil. Lead paint was also a significant problem many years ago. The peeling paint of older homes added lead to the soil around them. Many industries that produced metal products released high levels of contamination into both the air and the soil around factories.

Plants absorb heavy metals through their roots and to a lesser degree through their leaves. The amount they absorb depends on climate, the concentrations in soil, and the species of plant. Some plants are much better at picking up metals from soil than others, and these are generally called hyperaccumulators. When they are used to clean a contaminated site, the process is called phytoremediation.

A recent study tested a wide range of vegetables for their ability to absorb heavy metals and found that "the concentration of heavy metals in the edible parts of the vegetables decreased in the order of leafy vegetables > stalk vegetables/root vegetables/solanaceous vegetables > legume vegetables/melon vegetables." Leafy vegetables such as lettuce accumulated the most.[3]

Sunflower plants are very effective accumulators for nickel, copper, arsenic, lead, and especially cadmium, all of which ends up in both the seeds and sunflower oil. In the US, most confectionary sunflower seeds are grown in North and South Dakota, a region with relatively high cadmium levels in the soil. Strict rules in Europe have resulted in issues importing these products due to their high levels.

Breeders are now working to develop new cultivars that accumulate fewer heavy metals.

Dark chocolate is promoted as being healthy, but in recent years several reports have been published showing it contains heavy metals. Consumer Reports tested twenty-eight dark chocolate bars for lead and cadmium, and twenty-three of those violated California's maximum allowable dose levels (MADL) for lead or cadmium. It should be noted that California's MADL are higher than the rest of the country. Chocolate comes from the cocoa tree, which gets cadmium from the soil. Lead contamination happens after harvest when wet beans are exposed to soil and dust during the drying process.

Each crop absorbs heavy metals in different amounts. For example, rice naturally absorbs more arsenic, lettuce and onions accumulate lead more readily, and spinach and carrots accumulate cadmium more easily. Organically grown and non-GMO crops absorb just as much as other crops.

Although the above descriptions sound scary, the real risk from eating fruits and vegetables is very low, and the benefits far outweigh the risk. The presence of a hazard does not necessarily mean there is a risk. Most processed foods are tested for heavy metals and we can assume they meet government regulations. Fresh produce is not tested, and there is no easy way for a consumer to know the levels they are eating. There are, however, some things you can do in your garden to minimize exposure.

Control Heavy Metals in Your Garden

The largest potential source of contamination is your soil. If you live in a new development that was carved out of farmland or natural areas, you probably have little to be concerned about. On the other hand, if the home is in an old neighborhood, the soil might have gotten contaminated over the years. You can get your soil tested for heavy metals.

Older homes that have painted siding were probably painted with paint that contained lead. It is a good idea to test the soil to see if the levels are a concern.

Old raised beds made from either pressure-treated wood prior to about 2000 or old railway ties should be removed. Newer pressure-treated wood is safe for growing vegetables.

If testing shows that your soil is contaminated, you have two options for remediation: Remove the soil and replace it with clean soil, or grow super accumulators for a few years until testing shows a safe level. In the latter case, it is important to remove all vegetative growth from the property each year. Don't compost it, and don't keep it on the property.

Roads are also a potential source for heavy metals. Both car exhaust and small amounts of rubber from tires contain heavy metals. They travel through air and are washed onto neighboring soil when it rains. Gardens located near roads are potentially contaminated.

Airborne material is easily washed off produce and is not a serious problem. The amount of contamination in soil depends on the amount of traffic and the distance between the road and the garden. Highways are worse than local roads due to both the speed of the cars and the volume of traffic.

A Swedish study concluded that gardens are safe provided they are at least eighty feet away from a busy road, which is defined as three thousand cars per day. The move several years ago to low lead gasoline makes gardening near a road much safer. Growing food in front-yard gardens that are right next to quiet urban neighborhood streets is quite safe. If you live on a busy city street, it would be better to grow food in the backyard.

Each vegetable has a different ability to absorb heavy metals, and if there is a concern, you can select vegetables that are safer. Roots, leaves, and stems accumulate more than fruits (tomatoes, beans, etc.), so grow the fruits.

Low risk vegetables:

- tomatoes
- peppers
- beans
- zucchini

Moderate risk vegetables:

- cucumbers
- melons

High risk vegetables:

- potatoes
- carrots
- radishes
- onions
- collard greens
- Swiss chard
- lettuce

Food Safe Plastics

Growing food in plastic containers is on the rise, but there are potential risks if the wrong plastic is used. There are many different kinds of plastic, and even within a class of plastic there are variations. To help standardize this process, many are now given a recycle code along with an abbreviation for the plastic type. For example #1 is PET or PETE (polyethylene terephthalate).

Each type of plastic is made from different chemicals, has different properties, leaches different chemicals, and breaks down differently. Any general discussion about plastic and safety is of limited value if the plastic being discussed is not clearly defined.

All plastics leach chemicals, even the ones used for selling and storing food. The plastic water bottle, the plastic wrap around a salad, and even the plastic bag holding frozen vegetables leach chemicals. The difference between a safe plastic and one that is not safe is both the type and amount of chemical leached.

The plastic container used for growing food is filled with soil, watered, fertilized, and exposed to sun. Microbes in the soil decompose plastic, releasing chemicals. Contact with water and fertilizer also releases chemicals. Many plastics decompose in sunlight, adding more chemicals. These are all potentially absorbed by the plants.

Phthalates, often called plasticizers, are a group of chemicals of particular health concern and are absorbed by lettuce, strawberries, and carrots. Most of our exposure to plasticizers is from eating food, but we also inhale them and they are absorbed through our skin. The tolerable daily intake (TDI) has been set at 50 μg/kg body weight. They have been identified in most food groups, including fruits and vegetables. To put this into perspective, they have also been found in 252 cosmetic products (fragrances, hair sprays, deodorants, nail polishes, body lotions and creams, skin cleansers, and baby products). Your deodorant might be worse than the lettuce.

Bisphenol A (BPA) is found in polycarbonate plastic, which is used for containers to store food and beverages, such as water bottles. It can be toxic to plants at higher concentrations. BPA is not normally a problem in food grade plastics, but it, as well as lead, has been found in the new fabric pots.

Due to health concerns, BPA is sometimes replaced with two similar chemicals: BPS and BPAF. Testing of all three of these shows that BPA and BPS have a half-life of less than a day, so they don't last long in soil. BPAF has a half-life of about thirty days, which is still short compared to many other chemicals, but not nearly as good as for BPA.

The food safe grades of plastic includes #1, #2, #4, and #5. Most plastic containers have this number stamped on the bottom. If there is no number, you have no idea what kind of plastic it is.

Here are some examples I found around the house:

- peanut butter, ketchup, juice jars—all #1
- Tupperware—#5
- large Rubbermaid—#4
- 4" plant pot—#6 (polystyrene)

Types of food safe plastic and their code

- Home Depot 5 gallon pail—#2
- rain barrel (HDPE)—#2

Note that the 4" plant pot—which is designed for growing plants—is not food safe.

PVC (polyvinyl chloride, #3) is used a lot for water lines, and some people even grow food right in larger diameter pipes. It is especially popular for hydroponic growing. It is normally a hard plastic, but phthalates are added to make it softer and more flexible. It also contains some BPA. A form of PVC called uPVC or rigid PVC contains no phthalates and is considered food safe. It is best for the environment if you don't use regular PVC in the garden.

The other two non-food grade categories of plastic are #6 (polystyrene) and #7, which is used for any other plastic.

Much of the published information about plastic deals with it at normal room temperature and low light. In the garden, they are exposed to more heat and UV light from the sun. Both of these speed up chemical seepage and decomposition. Plastic can release BPA fifty times faster when in contact with boiling water than water at room temperature. PETE (#1) plastic will release the heavy metal antimony in the presence of heat. Polypropylene (#5) has a high heat tolerance, and tends to leach less than other plastics. How much of an effect does heat and sunlight have on plastics in the garden? The reality is that we don't know.

Is growing in plastic containers organic? You can grow in plastic and still be certified organic. That seems like a contradiction in terms to me. It is alright to grow in soil that contains chemicals from plastic, but is it not OK to use synthetic fertilizer, which is identical to the nutrients naturally released from soil? Even plastic mulch can be used in organic farming.

Growing in food grade plastic containers is considered safe.

Food safe plastics are also used in water drinking bottles and although they are considered safe, the plastic does leach out various chemicals into the water. The amount of such chemicals increases with time as the plastic degrades. It is the reason many people have switched to metal drinking bottles.

Problems with Plastic Mulch

Plastic mulch does a great job reducing weeds, and when used correctly it can increase yield. However, it also has issues.

Plastic mulch increases surface water runoff from both rainfall and irrigation. When pesticides are used, this runoff causes excess chemicals to move much more quickly into rivers and lakes, increasing pollution problems. Without the mulch, the chemicals seep into soil where many of them are decomposed by microbes before they enter waterways.

Chemical leaching is also a problem. Studies have shown that it leaches significant amounts of dibutyl phthalate, benzylbutyl phthalate, and acetyl tributyl citrate into soil.

The plastic also decomposes and adds microplastic particles into the soil, which can be picked up by the plants once they become nanoparticles.

US farms are generating nearly 860 million pounds of single use plastic waste annually, and almost none of it is recyclable.

Safe Material for Raised Beds

There is a strong trend toward using raised beds instead of growing in the ground. Some do it because they are concerned that the native soil might be contaminated, but except in special cases, this should not be a concern. Many build them so they don't have to bend down so much. The reality is that if you garden properly and use mulch, you do very little bending. A few minutes for planting. A few more minutes pulling out the odd weed or moving mulch to the side. Low crops such as beets and carrots require some bending for harvesting, but many crops are tall enough to harvest standing up. Unless you have physical disabilities, the benefits of a raised bed are limited. If you are a new gardener, I strongly suggest that you start by growing in the ground.

The material used for raised beds has the potential of contaminating the soil in the raised bed, and for this reason it should be selected with care.

Concrete Blocks

Concrete blocks are very popular for making raised beds. They produce a very solid wall, require no building experience, and are readily available. Unless you start adding concrete, you can't make the walls very high. A double row of bricks works well, and three high is probably the limit since taller walls are less stable. But a two-brick-high wall is more than adequate for most users. There are two concerns with concrete blocks: pH and heavy metals.

The pH of concrete is alkaline, and it is known that the soil around concrete foundations becomes alkaline as lime slowly seeps out. This might be a concern in very alkaline soil, but in most soil this is not a significant problem. In fact, many people add lime to acidic soil on a regular basis to raise the pH and sweeten the soil.

The second concern stems from the fact that fly ash is used to make concrete. Fly ash is the by-product of the coal industry and can contain heavy metals. Research has shown that the leaching of heavy metals from concrete is insignificant, and growing vegetables near concrete blocks is safe.

Untreated Wood

Wood is a good choice for raised beds. It is relatively inexpensive and can be used to make beds of various designs, and even tall walls are possible. They can also be fitted with sitting areas to make weeding easier.

Cheaper wood such as pine will last for six to eight years depending on climate. I use pine for my raised beds because I figure that in six years I will probably want to change things anyway. Cedar is much more expensive but lasts longer. Is this extra expense worth it? That depends on the price of cedar where you live.

There are no safety concerns with untreated wood.

Treated Wood

Cheap pine and other woods can be treated with chemicals to make them last as long as cedar. Prior to 2004, the chemicals used to make pressure-treated lumber included a process called CCA, which contained arsenic. Small amounts of arsenic can leach from this wood and be absorbed by plants. For this reason, CCA pressure-treated lumber is not recommended for raised beds.

Almost all of the pressure-treated lumber available today in North America and Europe uses a process called ACQ, which does not contain arsenic, but it does contain copper. ACQ treated wood is considered safe for use in the garden.

Certified organic production facilities are not allowed to use treated wood, but they are allowed to spray plants with copper fungicides—which are much more toxic than copper treated wood.

Cedar Wood

There is some concern among gardeners about the use of cedar for raised beds because of its allelopathic effects (explained below). It is important to understand which species of cedar we are talking about. There is the true cedar, which includes trees from the genus *Cedrus*, and the eastern red cedar (*Juniperus virginiana*), which is commonly called just cedar. There is also the western red cedar (*Thuja plicata*). The latter two are the most commonly used cedars to produce lumber.

J. virginiana has been shown to affect some seed germination and seedling growth; however, it does not affect most tested seed. Much of this testing is done in the lab, where wood extract is applied directly to the test soil. This is a more extreme treatment than using wood as the edge of a raised bed.

There is little evidence that cedar mulch has an effect on plant growth. Fresh cedar mulch can inhibit germination, but this effect is lost as the mulch ages. It is unlikely that using wood next to the soil will have any effect, even on seedlings.

Corrugated Metal

Corrugated metal is becoming a popular option because it is strong enough to make high beds at a reasonable cost. This material will last longer than wood, but to be honest, I think it looks ugly.

Corrugated metal is usually made from galvanized steel, which is coated with a zinc alloy. The zinc can leach out into the soil, but the levels are very small. Both plants and animals require some zinc in their diet, so there is no health concern.

Microplastics

Microplastics are very small particles of plastic that are less than 0.2 inches (5 mm) in length. They are created as plastic degrades. In the environment, microplastics keep breaking up into smaller and smaller pieces, eventually forming nanoplastic particles. The process is slow, but even very tiny pieces can impact the environment.

Food itself is also a source of microplastic particles. A recent study found three hundred thousand pieces of microplastics per kilogram of food waste collected from grocery stores in the United States. Even bottled water contained 325 particles per liter.

The research looking at the effect of these small particles on food production and soil is limited but ongoing. Plants do absorb nanoplastic particles into roots and these have been found in the edible portion of food, with roots having higher levels than above-ground vegetables. Plastic particles can affect the properties of soil, including texture and structure, which in turn may impact plant performance.[4]

Growing Food Near Toxic Plants

A number of common garden plants are toxic, including lily of the valley, hyacinths, daffodils, monkshood, oleander, foxglove, and delphinium to name a few. Some weeds, such as hemlock, are also poisonous. These plants exude chemicals into the soil through their roots, and falling leaves get incorporated into the soil. What happens when food plants are grown in this soil?

The amount of toxins in soil from plants is very small. Most of these compounds become a food source for microbes, which further decreases the amount. In order for another plant to pick up toxins it needs to absorb it through their roots, and that won't happen for most larger molecules. Even if absorbed, the enzymes in the plant will likely dispose of it. The transfer of poisons from one plant to another is not an issue, but there are some other things to consider.

Sweet peas are toxic to humans, while garden peas are not. The problem is that both plants produce similar-looking pods. It would be quite easy for an inexperienced gardener, or a child, to mistake one for the other and eat toxic peas.

Growing daffodils next to your onions can pose a similar problem. I think they look quite different, and they grow at different depths, but if you are harvesting in a hurry, or an animal has dug up a daffodil bulb, you might mistake the two.

Some people are also concerned about poison hemlock (*Conium maculate*) which is an invasive, noxious weed, and all parts of the plant are poisonous. Having this plant in the garden will not result in poison being transferred to vegetables. However, it is important that you do not confuse its roots with parsnip and parsley.[5]

All parts of a potato, except the tuber, are poisonous and yet nobody suggests keeping them outside of the vegetable garden. It is probably best not to grow toxic plants in a vegetable garden, but there is no risk of your food becoming toxic.

Allelopathy

Allelopathy is a biological phenomenon where an organism produces chemicals that affect the growth and survival of another organism. Allelochemicals can have beneficial or detrimental consequences. In the strict definition this applies to any type of organism, but the term is commonly used by gardeners to describe interactions between plants and most of the discussion centers around detrimental effects.

The most well-known case of allelopathy is the effect walnut trees have on the growth of other plants. It is believed by many that nothing grows under a walnut tree because it excretes a chemical called juglone.

The reality of this story is quite different. The various parts of a walnut tree don't contain any juglone. They do have another compound that turns into juglone on exposure to air, but this quickly converts to even more compounds. Juglone will prevent some seedlings, notably tomatoes and other nightshades, from growing, but most of the studies showing this have been done in the lab and not the real world.

Nobody has been able to demonstrate that plant roots actually take up juglone from the soil. If they don't absorb it, how can it affect plant growth? It is true that some plants don't grow as well under a walnut tree, but most mature plants grow just fine.

Other examples of allelopathy include garlic mustard (*Alliaria petiolate*), which inhibits the growth of other plants and mycorrhizal fungi. Mexican fireweed (*Bassia scoparia*), an invasive weed in central North America, reduces the growth of spring wheat.

There are many other claims of plant-to-plant allelopathy, but most of the details of these are not well understood. The chemical effects of allelopathy reach beyond the rhizosphere, but weaken as one gets farther away from plant roots. I suspect the effect is real, but not nearly as potent as claimed in gardening circles.

Another plant that has been shown to be allelopathic is the sunflower. Field studies have found that the presence of a preceding sunflower crop decreased plant height, dry matter, and yield of subsequent crops, including sorghum, pearl millet, maize, cotton, sunflowers, cluster beans, cowpeas, and green gram. Future sunflower crops were affected more than most other crops.

If you have a choice, don't put your vegetable garden near walnut trees. If that is the only location you have, focus on growing plants that are not affected by juglone, such as lima and snap beans, beets, corn, onions, garlic, leeks, parsnip, carrots, cauliflower, parsley, Jerusalem artichoke, melons, and squash. Avoid planting vegetables that are sensitive to juglone, such as asparagus, cabbage, eggplant, peas, peppers, potatoes, rhubarb, and tomatoes. This latter group can be grown in raised beds that have a bottom that will keep walnut roots out of the soil, or in containers.

GMO Food

About 89 percent of scientists agree that GMO food is safe, while 57 percent of Americans say GMO food is *not* safe. This drastic disconnect is both interesting and troubling. The difference may be due to the fact that people do not trust science, or that the anti-GMO movement has done a really good job of brainwashing the public. It is probably a bit of both.[6]

Lots of seed catalogs selling to gardeners promote the idea that their seed is "GMO free." That is deceptive marketing because all seed sold to home gardeners, with one exception, is GMO free. In fact, most of the vegetables we grow don't even exist as GMO seeds. The only GMO fruits and vegetables available in the US are corn, potato, papaya, apple, pink pineapple, and summer squash, and these are only sold to farmers who sign a contract and who buy larger quantities. This is not a gardening issue.

The first GMO vegetable was made available to home gardeners in 2024. It is a tomato called 'Purple' and was only made available in the US through Norfolk Healthy Products. It contains higher levels of anthocyanin, which makes it very purple both inside and outside. Anthocyanin is the antioxidant that makes blueberries a superfood.

Most GMO crops grown in the US are used to make processed food or animal feed. A few items such as potato, papaya, apple, pink pineapple, and summer squash are available as GMO produce, but only papaya is commonly found.

Many people fear GMO mostly because they don't understand it. If you equate GMO with Roundup or Monsanto, you have been misinformed.

GMO is a technology for making new cultivars. Scientists in a lab are able to move genes from one organism into another in order to give the new plant special characteristics. We call this new plant a "genetically modified organism." They are commonly called a GMO plant, but the term should really only be used for the technology. The reason for this is that we now have newer technology such as CRISPR that also makes genetically modified organisms, but does not use GMO technology.

Did you know that the sweet potato is a naturally formed genetically modified organism? When scientists studied the DNA of the sweet potato, they found that it contained DNA from a bacteria genus called *Agrobacterium*, and this DNA has been there for thousands of years. *Agrobacterium* uses a method of transferring its DNA into other species that is very similar to the method used to make GMOs. The sweet potato has DNA from both plants and bacteria and is a natural GMO produced by nature. Should the sweet potato be called a GMO?[7]

The ringspot virus disease nearly wiped out Hawaii's papaya crop by the 1990s. A GMO variety, called Rainbow papaya, was created to resist the virus, and this new variety saved the papaya industry on the Hawaiian Islands.

Rice is a main staple of many developing countries, and although it provides energy and minerals, it is very low in vitamins. A deficiency of vitamin A in the diet is responsible for a million deaths annually, most of them children, plus an additional five hundred thousand cases of blindness. A special GMO rice called Golden Rice was produced that contains high levels of beta-carotene, which the body converts into vitamin A. The beta-carotene gives the rice grains its yellowish color, which inspired its name. The seed for this rice has been made available free of charge on a global basis, but all the political, ideological, and emotional baggage that is associated with GMOs has kept many countries from using it.[8]

Did you take the COVID vaccine? It was produced with a newer form of GMO technology. These proved extremely valuable, and the genetic modification produced no side effects. It did not, as some claim, turn us into genetically modified organisms.

Is GMO Food Safe to Eat?

There is absolutely no scientific evidence that GMO food is harmful to eat. You might be surprised at that statement since the anti-GMO movement continues to display pictures of rats with tumors from a study done years ago by Gilles-Eric Séralini. This work has been completely debunked and the author was forced to withdraw the work because it was so poorly done.

Consider this for a moment. GMO technique moves a couple of very specific genes from one organism to another. The process is very controlled; the scientists know exactly which genes are being moved, and the DNA in the resulting organism is well tested. Compare that to natural plant breeding where you mix and shake thousands of genes, have no idea what is in the new organism, and do almost no testing. And yet natural plant breeding this is considered to be perfectly safe to eat.

GMO technology and the food produced from it is perfectly safe to eat. In fact, it is much safer than traditional breeding of plants, and it is safer than other technologies such as mutagenesis, although neither of these alternatives are high risk.

The Future of Genetically Modified Food

The tools we have today are even better than those of only a few years ago. We can now accurately edit a single base unit in DNA. What this means is that scientists can change DNA in very precise ways. This makes the process thousands of times safer than traditional breeding.

Scientists are working on crops that will give higher yields with the same amount of fertilizer and fewer pesticides. They are creating plants that fix nitrogen from the air so that they need much less fertilizer. Climate change will make the planet warmer and in some regions drier. New crops are on the way that will grow in such dry conditions. Other crops are being developed to be much more salt tolerant so that we can use salty soil and irrigation water. Plants can be modified so that they produce more nutrients, making them more nutritious. GMO has led to the meatless burger, the Arctic apple that resists browning, and vanilla flavoring produced by yeast.

Genetic manipulation of plants, especially for food crops, is here to stay and as the saying goes, you ain't seen nothing yet.

Allergies and Sensitivities

Food allergies and sensitivities are illnesses that affect only certain individuals, compared to other types of foodborne illness that affect everyone. Many consumers, and even health professionals, use the term "allergy" to incorrectly refer to both allergies and sensitivities. Many consumers also believe they have one or the other of these conditions without a proper medical diagnosis. In one study, only 25 percent of the people with self-reported gluten sensitivity had the right symptoms for the disease. Thirty percent of Americans avoid gluten because of sensitivities, while only 1 percent of the population has celiac disease.

Food allergies are abnormal immunological reactions to a particular food or substance in a food. This reaction releases antibodies and causes the body to react as if it is threatened. A lot of times this is caused by naturally occurring proteins, and even small amounts can cause severe life-threatening reactions. Responses can be immediate, taking a few minutes or be delayed, in which case they take forty-eight to seventy-two hours to manifest themselves.

Ninety percent of allergic reactions are caused by milk, eggs, fish, shellfish, peanuts, tree nuts, wheat, and soybeans. People who are allergic to these foods must avoid even small quantities of them. A severe reaction is known as anaphylaxis and can cause a significant drop in blood pressure, leading to fainting and loss of consciousness.

Food intolerances are not immune responses. They often trigger a reaction in the digestive system or gastrointestinal tract, resulting in stomach upset and discomfort. Symptoms are not life-threatening and can include gas, bloating, diarrhea, constipation, cramping, and nausea. For example, lactose intolerance is when your body can't break down lactose properly.

Legumes such as soy, peanuts, beans, and chickpeas can cause both intolerance and allergic reactions. An allergic condition is due to a reaction to the proteins found in legumes, but it is not very common. An intolerance to legumes is caused by the fibers in the food. They are difficult for us to digest, and bacteria help this process. While they feed on the starches, they produce gasses which cause discomfort as your belly distends. The starches also draw water into the intestines, causing you to feel full and have loose bowel movements.

Peanuts are not a true legume because they are not seeds, although they are produced on a plant in the legume family.

4
Food Safety—Biological

Biological food safety deals with the effect of living organisms on our health. You can't see them because they are microscopic, but all food is covered with microbes. Even freshly washed food has microbes on it and the longer the food sits, the more microbes it accumulates both from the air and because they can reproduce rapidly. Not to worry—your hands may be covered with more microbes than your food.

If microbes are everywhere, why are we not sick all of the time? Most microbes do not harm us and our body defenses are quite good at dealing with minor infections. However, this does not mean that we should be complacent about them. Some can make us sick, and there are many things we can do to limit their effect.

The symptoms of food poisoning depend on the organism causing it, but the most common symptoms are nausea and diarrhea. Not everyone will necessarily get food poisoning even if they eat the same thing. In healthy individuals, stomach acid kills food poisoning bacteria, while lactic acid bacteria in the intestines create an environment that is inhospitable to problem bacteria.

People with relatively weak immune systems (low resistance to disease) such as children, senior citizens, and adults with weakened immune systems can get food poisoning more easily. In addition, the time required for symptoms to show themselves as well as the strength of the symptoms can vary depending on the amount of bacteria ingested.

Bacteria that cause food poisoning can be detected in the stool of a person even if they show no symptoms. Such "healthy carriers" can unknowingly contaminate food with bacteria and viruses such as the highly infectious Enterohemorrhagic *E. coli* and norovirus, spreading them to others and causing an outbreak of food poisoning. If your family gets food poisoning and you don't have any symptoms, you may be a healthy carrier. Take care not to spread the disease by washing your hands thoroughly with soap and water after going to the bathroom.

Most common types of food poisoning will take four to twenty-four hours to set in, but it's not always that quick. Some foodborne illnesses are latent, meaning they reproduce in your system before you feel any symptoms. The virus hepatitis A, for example, can take fifteen to fifty days before rearing its ugly head.

Most of the time, symptoms pass within twelve to forty-eight hours in healthy people, but it can vary based on several factors and in some cases it can last ten days or more. For example, symptoms from the bacteria *Campylobacter* can last for weeks. Talk with your doctor if your symptoms last longer than two days.

The Microbes Among Us

The main microbes that cause a biological hazard include bacteria, viruses, fungi, and parasites. I have described these extensively in my book *Microbe Science for Gardeners*, so this section will just give a brief overview.

Bacteria

Bacteria need the following to grow: nitrogen, moisture, pH above 4.5, oxygen, and an acceptable temperature. Given the right conditions, bacteria grow at exponential rates, and that is why it is so important to prevent growth before they get started.

Viruses

Unlike bacteria, viruses do not grow in food, but they can stay viable until eaten and then infect us.

Fungi, Mold, Yeast

Molds are a type of fungi, as are yeast. Mold itself is not a problem if it is ingested, but the chemicals mold produces can be quite toxic. Yeast can cause pink patches on moist cheese or cloudiness in condiments such as olives, but it does not cause illness.

Parasites

Parasites are tiny organisms that can cause disease. *Cryptosporidium* and *Giardia* are two examples of these. Cooking will normally kill them.

What Is a Foodborne Illness

For the most part, microbes do not harm us. Your gut contains more bacteria than all the cells in your body and they are not only good for you, they are actually essential to help you digest food. Unfortunately, there are a few microbes that can harm us, and when they do, we generally call it a foodborne illness. Other terms used for this include foodborne infection, food intoxication, food poisoning, and some call it a disease. The term illness implies that it is a disease, but that is not a very good term because it is either an infection or a poisoning.

No matter what you call it, it can be very serious. One in six Americans will develop a foodborne illness each year (17 percent). This number should almost certainly be higher since most people do not report it. The CDC reports that of these, 128,000 will end up in hospital and 3,000 will die.[1]

Microbes can make us sick in one of three ways: intoxication, infection, or toxicoinfection.

Intoxication results when we ingest toxic compounds produced by the microbes. Two of the most commonly cited bacteria include *Staphylococcus aureus* and *Clostridium botulinum*, as well as a common mold called *Aspergillus flavus*. In these cases, the microbe itself does not harm us. It is the chemicals the microbes excrete that are toxic to us.

The microbes that cause intoxication do not need to be alive to cause a problem. For example, if you cook some contaminated meat and kill all of the microbes, the remaining toxin can still make you sick.

Infection happens when you ingest live microbes that then grow in your gut, resulting in illness. Bacteria that cause infection include *Salmonella enterica*, *Campylobacter jejuni*, *Escherichia coli*, and *Listeria monocytogenes*. Hepatitis A and Norovirus are also in this group.

Toxicoinfection, also called toxin-mediated infection, is an illness where the ingestion of large amounts of microbes produce a toxin after they are ingested. *Clostridium perfringens*, *Bacillus cereus*, and *E. coli* are examples.

In all three of the above cases, the effect is felt in our GI tract, so symptoms include nausea, vomiting, abdominal cramps, diarrhea, and maybe fever. Each person reacts differently to the same contaminated food. Some will become seriously ill, while others show no symptoms at all.

The important take-home message is that both living and dead microbes can cause foodborne illness. Preventing this type of illness comes down to eliminating the presence of microbes before we eat the food and preventing them from growing in the first place. Even dead microbes can harm you.

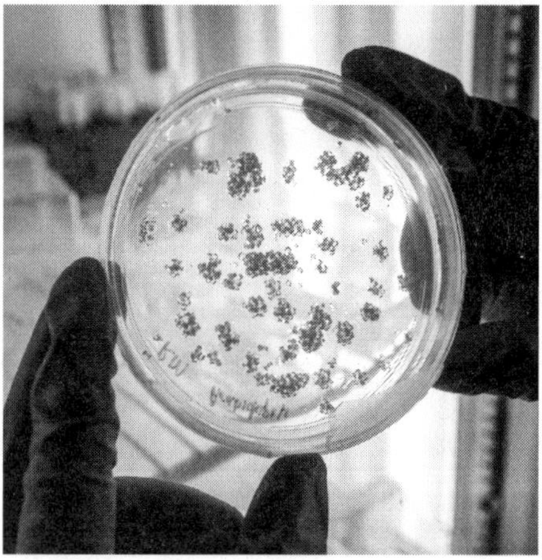

Microbes growing in a petri dish
Credit: DOE Joint Genome Institute[2]

How Microbes Grow

It is important to understand that microbes represent hundreds of thousands of different species and each one has different requirements for life. They prefer different temperatures, different foods, and even different gasses in the air. Understanding their needs will help you control them. These environmental factors can be divided into two groups: the nature of the actual food, known as the intrinsic factors, and the storage environment around the food, the extrinsic factors.

Intrinsic food factors include the following:

- type of food
- pH
- availability of water
- oxygen
- antimicrobials (essential oils in spices, enzymes in eggs and milk)
- physical structures (shells, skins, hides)

Extrinsic storage factors include the following:

- temperature
- relative humidity
- inhibitory gasses (CO_2, ozone)
- other organisms

Too much or too little of any factor will slow down growth or even kill the microbe. Some of these factors can have cumulative negating effects. For example, dry conditions make it difficult for bacteria to survive. Combine that with high temperatures and they die even faster. Many of these factors can be controlled during food storage and food preparation, so it is important to understand how each affects microbes.

What happens to the bacterial population when conditions change? If the changes are negative, bacteria either go dormant—a kind of hibernation—or they die. When conditions become more favorable, they grow at a very fast rate. This growth follows the bacterial growth curve pictured below.

The lag phase represents the time before any change in conditions. There is a steady number of bacteria. As conditions improve, bacteria enter the exponential phase where the number increases quickly. At some point, this growth becomes a negative factor because food runs out, toxins build up, and oxygen levels decrease—it is just too crowded for more growth. The population then enters the death phase where bacteria start to die off, eventually returning to a lag phase.

For food safety, it is important to prevent the exponential phase from ever happening.

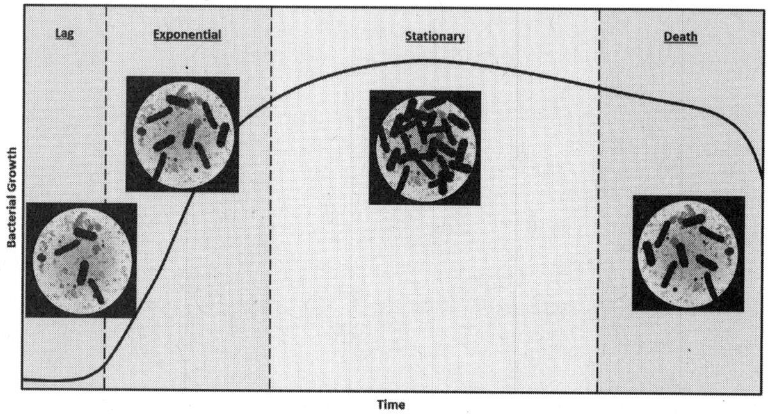

Growth of bacteria over time

pH

pH is the measure of acidity and uses a scale from zero to fourteen, with seven being neutral. Anything below seven is acidic, and a substance becomes more acidic as the pH gets smaller. Values above seven indicate an alkaline or "basic" condition.

Each microbe has a preferred pH range and if the pH gets too high or too low, their growth will suffer, and at extremes they will die. Some bacteria and fungi (acidophiles) like acid conditions and can even live in lemon juice and gastric acids at pH 2. The alkaliphiles like the alkaline conditions found in soda lakes and alkaline soil. Most prefer a more neutral pH between five and nine.

Processes such as pickling and fermentation take advantage of the fact that most pathogens can't survive at low pH. For this reason, it is important to follow directions exactly when using any preservation methods that lower pH.

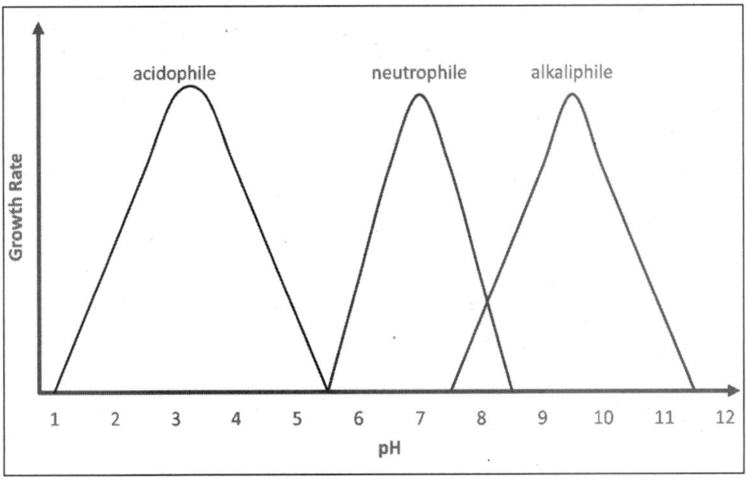

Preferred pH range for bacterial groups

Water

We talk about bacteria living on solid surfaces such as vegetables and tabletops or in soil, but the reality is that most of them need to live in water. Since they are so small, this can be a very thin film of water, but they will die without water.

It is important to understand the difference between bound and unbound water. Bound water consists of water molecules that are tied up with things such as sugar or cell structures so that bacteria can't use it. If you take an apple and squeeze the water out, the water that comes out is unbound water. The remaining pulp might seem dry, but it still contains some water that is bound to other molecules and the remaining cell structure. This bound water is not available to bacteria.

Molds need more water than yeast, which need more water than bacteria. The process of drying meat, fish, and fruits results in food that has no unbound water and is therefore a poor place for microbes to grow. Adding large amounts of sugar to water also ties up the water and prevents microbial growth.

Humidity

Imagine going into a damp, warm root cellar in summer. That musty smell is from the growth of microbes, mainly molds, which are fungi. Microbes grow better at high humidity, which is no surprise since humidity is just water moisture in the air, and microbes need water.

High humidity keeps microbes from drying out by creating a moist layer right next to their exterior cell walls. Increasing the humidity from 50 to 70 percent relative humidity increases bacterial growth by 2.8 times and an increase to 90 percent relative humidity increases growth by 6.2 times.

Oxygen

Microbes can be divided into three categories based on their need for oxygen. The aerobes need oxygen and can't live long without it. Many of these microbes are beneficial. At the other extreme you find organisms that grow best at low levels of oxygen, and many of these are pathogens. Microbes that can live in both environments are called facultative anaerobes. *E. coli* is a common example of a facultative bacteria that can live both on the surface of food where there is lots of oxygen and in our intestine, which has low levels of oxygen.

Vacuum packing food removes the air and thus the oxygen, resulting in an environment where many food-spoiling bacteria can't grow because they are aerobes. This kind of packaging does increase the risk of growing anaerobes. This is a common packing technique for cheese, cured meats, fish, ground coffee, cereals, nuts, and pasta.

Temperature

Bacteria can exist in a very wide range of temperatures. They exist everywhere on Earth, including the arctic, deserts, and in hot springs. However, each species has a preferred temperature range. As temperatures go outside of this range, bacteria either die or go into a state of hibernation called dormancy. In the dormant stage, they can survive more extreme temperatures. Other types of microbes tend to be more demanding for their preferred range.

Temperature has a dramatic effect on growth rate. The bacteria in milk grow quite quickly at room temperature, but very slowly in the fridge. But milk will eventually sour even at lower temperatures due to bacteria growth.

Most microbes that cause foodborne illness tend to be mesophiles that prefer temperatures around 102°F (39°C). Some species have different strains for different temperatures, allowing them to exist in a wide range. *E. coli*, for example, grows in a range of 46°F to 118°F (8°C to 48°C).

Bacteria grow fastest in the range of 40°F to 140°F (4°C to 60°C), where they can double in number every twenty minutes. This range is called the "danger zone." This is why self-serve restaurants use both a cold bar and a hot bar to keep food outside of this range and health experts caution people not to keep meat outside of the refrigerator for more than two hours.

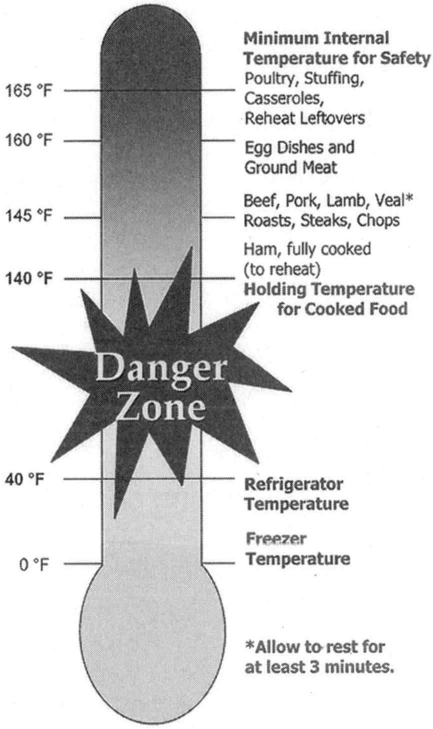

Bacteria grow fastest in the "Danger Zone"
Credit: USDA Food Safety and Inspection Service [3]

A doubling time of twenty minutes may not seem too significant, but consider this: A single bacterium doubling at this rate for forty-eight hours would create a mass that is more than the mass of all the planets in our solar system. Of course this does not happen because in the real world, the doubling rate is slower when conditions are not perfect and the bacteria soon run out of food, which stops growth.[4]

Here is a more realistic example: Your chicken casserole has forty salmonella cells per gram when you take it out of the fridge. After sitting on the picnic table for four hours at 90°F (32°C), it will contain 2,621,440 cells per gram, or one billion per 350 g serving. As few as one hundred thousand salmonella cells can make you sick.

Detecting a Problem

How do you know if food is contaminated with microbes? Unfortunately, you have no easy way to tell. For the most part, microbes are small and invisible to our eyes, but there are some things you can do.

The best thing you can do is to use your eyes, nose, and touch. Look for abnormal coloration, colored growths, or soft spots. Green fuzzy fungal growth is easy to spot. Feel the texture. A slimy feel is almost certainly due to a bacterial party. A bad smell or sour smell can also indicate microbes. Some of these indicators may just be due to spoiled food, but usually spoilage is accompanied by microbial growth.

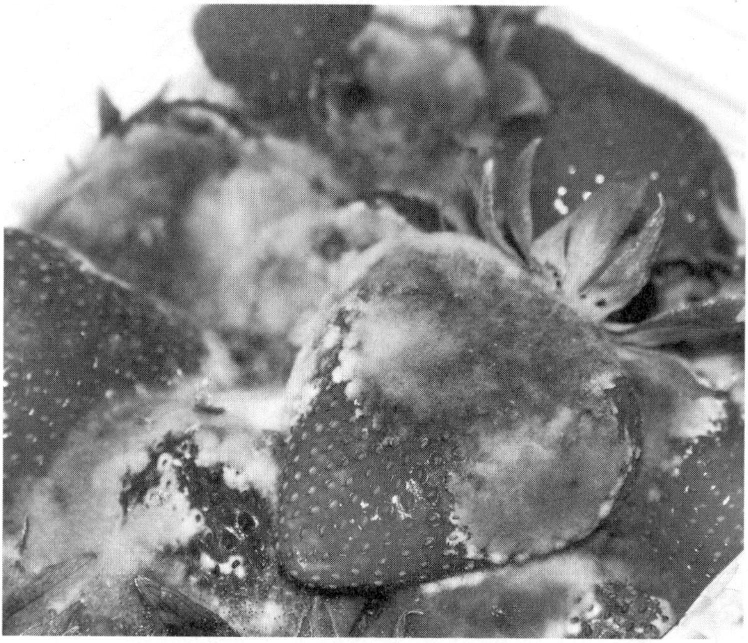

Use sight and smell to detect microbes Credit: Casey Bisson [5]

Meaning of "Best if Used By" Date

Food can be labeled with a number of dates including "best if used by," "best before," "expiry," or "use-by date." A common belief is that these dates indicate food safety, meaning that food that is past these dates should not be used because the risk of biological contamination is too high. As a result, such food is thrown out and that is a big waste of usable food.

These dates have nothing to do with food safety. The dates indicate food quality. The manufacturer or packager determines the date when the quality may not be at its "best." In most cases, there is nothing wrong with eating food that has exceeded these dates, provided it was stored properly.

Fruit Browning

Bruising or cutting some fruits and vegetables results in flesh turning brown. This happens in apples, apricots, bananas, cherries, peaches, pears, eggplant, and potatoes. An enzyme called polyphenol oxidase in the damaged flesh is exposed to higher levels of oxygen from the air, which causes it to react with phenolic compounds, producing brown melanins. This process is called "enzymatic browning." You might be familiar with the term melanin, the pigment that gives human hair, skin, and eyes their color.

This brown material is unsightly, but there are no health concerns with it. It is perfectly fine to eat. Enzymatic browning is controlled by reducing the oxygen. One solution is to cover the fruit with a sugar syrup, which keeps out oxygen. This is effectively used in making jam. Acids, including citric acid powder, ascorbic acid, and lemon juice work by reducing the pH to where the enzyme can't function. Low temperatures, freezing, and high temperatures slow down or damage the enzyme and also prevent browning. Blanching also works since the short exposure to boiling water is enough to destroy the enzyme.

The Arctic apple is a GMO apple that is nonbrowning when cut. Currently, food service companies that want to include cut apples need to treat them with antioxidant chemicals such as calcium ascorbate to keep them looking fresh, but this will no longer be needed with the Arctic apple. In this case, extra copies of genes that are naturally found in apples were inserted into the DNA. The new apple produces less polyphenol oxidase, resulting in less browning.

You might not like the brown color on your apple, but this same reaction is also responsible for some of the color and taste in coffee, tea, and chocolate. Next time your apple goes brown, just think of it as being coated in chocolate—problem solved.

Buying Food

Keeping food safe starts with growing it properly, or buying safe food. Here are some things you can do to reduce the risk of buying contaminated food:

- be mindful of the danger zone and pick the hot and cold items at the end of the shopping trip
- keep the frozen items at one end of your cart so they stay colder and place that hot barbecued chicken at the other end
- put all the cold items in the same shopping bag and the hot in a different bag
- don't buy swollen, dented, or leaking cans
- don't buy ready-to-eat foods left uncovered on counters
- check that serving staff wear gloves when handling food and then take them off when they clean surfaces or handle money
- never buy cracked or dirty eggs—check the carton every time
- take your shopping home quickly and get it into the fridge right away
- use a cooler for longer shopping trips

Food Safety Myths

The CDC has reported that 46 percent of all foodborne illnesses are due to fresh produce, and one out of every six Americans will get a foodborne illness this year. Fresh produce was linked to less than 1 percent of all foodborne illnesses in the 1970s, and less than 12 percent in the 1990s. There has been a significant increase since then.[6]

Part of the increase is due to better detection, but it is also due to increased use of fast food and a more complex food production/delivery system. Food that we buy in local stores has passed through many hands from farm to table, and each step is a possible source of contamination. Another problem is that more people are growing their own food and they incorrectly believe that homegrown food is safe.

The following are some myths about foodborne illnesses and how you can prevent them:

Myth #1: Unsafe Food Smells Bad

Microbes make food spoil, and as part of this process they create compounds that smell. This is a different group of organisms than the ones that make you ill, and most spoiled food is not an ideal environment for pathogens that make you sick. You can't detect pathogens by smell. It is still not a good idea to eat spoiled food.

Myth #2: You Can't Catch a Foodborne Illness

People do spread some of these pathogens. For example, you can catch hepatitis A from another person through fecal-oral transmission. That is exactly what it sounds like: someone did not wash their hands properly after having a crap. It is more common than you think.

Myth #3: Washing Produce with Soap Makes It Safe

Using soap or detergent to wash produce is not safe because the chemicals stick to food and are not safe for consumption. Not only that, but they don't remove pathogens any better than clean running water.

Myth #4: Peeling Removes Pathogens

Peeling is not much better than washing. Microbes on the outside of produce easily travel to the newly exposed surfaces through contact with hands and knives. The process of peeling also damages the surface of the remaining tissue, making it easy for pathogens to gain entry into the flesh of produce where they have access to released nutrients, making a perfect environment for pathogens to grow. Don't peel produce until you are ready to cook it, or eat it raw.

Myth #5: Organic Produce Has More Pathogens

The perception is that organic farmers are more likely to use manure, which is seen as a source of pathogens. The reality is that both organic and conventional agriculture use manure, but organic use is more regulated, which should reduce pathogens. There are only a few studies that have compared pathogens in the two forms of farming and they have found no differences in the level of pathogens on the produced food. Organically certified farms may actually produce food with fewer pathogens.

Manure use is safe provided it is hot composted (at least 131°F (55°C) or it is buried in soil well in advance of planting. Reported cases of illness resulting from the use of raw manure are very rare.

Myth #6: Pesticides Kill Pathogens

Some people believe that conventionally grown food is safer because it has been treated with pesticides that kill the pathogens along with the pest. First of all, both organic and conventional food can be sprayed with pesticides. Secondly, most pesticides don't kill bacteria.

Spraying with pesticides might even increase the level of pathogens because the water used to mix up the pesticide is usually non-potable water that contains microbes. Some of the pesticides are a food source for microbes, causing microbes to grow in holding tanks. This problem has been identified as a source of foodborne illness and is being targeted with new regulations. Home gardeners should use municipal water when mixing pesticides, including DIY remedies, and the mixed solutions should not be stored for future use.

Myth #7: Vegetarians Don't Have to Worry About Food Poisoning

It is a common belief that food poisoning is mostly the result of eating contaminated meat, but fruits and vegetables are just as likely to make you sick. Leafy greens have been a regular source of illness and need to be washed very well.

Myth #8: Freezing Food Kills Harmful Bacteria

Bacteria can survive freezing. The lower temperature does slow their growth significantly, but freezing does not make your food safe. As food thaws, bacteria come out of dormancy and start to multiply. That is one reason defrosting food on a warm kitchen counter is not a good idea. It is better to do it in the fridge, or quickly in cold water. Once food is thawed, keep it in the fridge until you are ready to cook it.

Viruses, such as hepatitis A, can survive freezing, freeze-drying, and heat of less than 185°F (85°C). A recent outbreak of hepatitis from frozen berries is a good example of this.

Myth #9: Microwaving Food Kills the Bacteria

Microwaves do not kill bacteria. They energize water molecules, resulting in heat. Bacteria are killed by high temperatures. Microwaved food tends to heat unevenly, even with a turntable, and so sections of food that don't get hot enough will still contain live bacteria.

Myth #10: Moldy Food Is OK to Eat

Maybe. Mold itself is usually not harmful if eaten, but the growing mold may produce mycotoxins, which can make you sick. Remember that mold produces root-like structures that go deep into food—it is not just the fuzzy stuff you see on the outside. If you see mold, it is very likely that bacteria are also growing in the same spot.

On the other hand, some mold is good for you. Penicillin is made from mold, and the fungi *Penicillium camemberti* is responsible for the production of camembert and brie.

Myth #11: I Don't Have Pathogens in My Garden

Even if you don't use manure and don't have pets, your garden does have pathogens. Every garden has birds, insects, and animals using the garden as a toilet, and they all add pathogens. Even that organic soil you have contains human pathogens such as *Listeria monocytogenes* and *Clostridium botulinum* (producing botulin toxin). Water from a rain barrel, compost tea, and weed tea are all contaminated to some extent.

You should assume everything in the garden is a potential source of human pathogens. It's one reason for washing your hands after being in the garden.

Myth #12: Hot Compost Is Pathogen Free

From my book *Compost Science for Gardeners*: "Pathogens are killed by heat and time. At 115°F (46°C) pathogens are killed off in a week, while at 144°F (62°C) they are killed off in an hour." The problem with home compost piles is that they rarely get hot enough to kill off the pathogens, and even if they are killed off, more will arrive in the compost during the curing process. Remember that pathogens are found everywhere in the garden. That does not mean you should stop using compost because the benefits far outweigh the risks.

Myth #13: Water From a Rain Barrel Is Pathogen Free

Collected rain water can contain pathogens, but it is not a significant source if the water is used properly. For more on this and other myths about water collected in rain barrels, see *Myths About Rainwater Harvesting Systems for Gardens*.[7]

Final Thoughts

Foodborne illness is important and can be serious, but it should not be a major source of concern. Follow good hygiene practices. Wash your hands after gardening. Wash any produce you bring into the house, both from the garden and the store. When possible, keep the food cold to slow microbial growth.

What about eating that fresh strawberry or tomato right in the garden? It is not recommended, but almost all gardeners do it and live to tell about it. You are now a risk taker!

5

Nutrient Density

What is nutrient density? Also called biodensity, the National Cancer Institute defines it this way: "Food that is high in nutrients but relatively low in calories. Nutrient-dense foods contain vitamins, minerals, complex carbohydrates, lean protein, and healthy fats."

That seems like a logical definition, but doesn't all produce contain vitamins, minerals, complex carbohydrates, lean protein, and healthy fats (or oils)? Sure they do. By this definition, all fruits and vegetables are nutrient dense, but that's not much help.

The US Department of Agriculture defines a nutrient-rich food index (NRF) based on nine nutrients that should be consumed (protein; fiber; vitamins A, C, and E; calcium; iron; potassium; and magnesium) and three nutrients that should be avoided (saturated fat, added sugar, and sodium). The idea behind NRF is to eat fewer calories and still get high amounts of the things your body needs. But what about all the other things in food, such as antioxidants and phytochemicals? They are also important.

Without going into this in more detail, there is no single accepted definition for nutrient-dense food. Several new systems, such as nutrient profiling, are being developed because all of the current systems have flaws. Remember that vegetables contain thousands of chemicals and in many cases we still don't know what role they play in our health. Without that knowledge, it is really impossible to define which nutrients are most important to us.

Let me illustrate the problems with these systems. A slice of white bread contains about 100 micrograms of vitamin E, and a slice of brown bread contains 350 micrograms. Many would conclude that the brown bread is more nutrient dense because it has more vitamin E. But what if the white bread had a higher level of calcium? Which one is more nutrient dense?

Some consider salmon to be a high nutrient-dense food because a 3.5 ounce (100 gram) piece of wild salmon contains 0.1 ounces (2.8 g) of omega-3. But omega-3 is not even one of the nutrients considered important in the above NRF index.

Once a fruit or vegetable is picked, its vitamin C content starts to drop and for this reason fresh vegetables are considered to have a higher nutrient density. However, the average person in North America already gets enough vitamin C in their diet. Eating food with higher levels of vitamin C are of little value since the excess is just excreted from the body. So should vitamin C even be counted when measuring nutrient density?

Should nutrient density not rather focus on the nutrients that are in short supply in our bodies? If we get enough vitamin C and calcium, does it not make sense to ignore these nutrients when we are trying to quantify the nutritional value of a food?

These are just some of the problems with defining nutrient-dense food, and if we can't clearly define it, how can gardeners expect to grow food with a higher nutrient density?

My personal opinion is that the term is not understood by most of the people using it, and therefore all kinds of misinformation has been spread by its use. We can't compare two food items and categorically identify the most nutritious one. We can test two apples and say one apple has more vitamin C than the other apple, but that does not make it more nutritious.

Measuring Nutrient Density

The term nutrient density is not well defined, but the concept is valid. We want to grow and consume the most nutritious food we can. In order to do that, we need to be able to measure nutrition. If you can't measure it or get a number off a label, it is impossible to make the best choice.

Have you ever seen a nutrient density number on any food you buy? I haven't either. Without that number, you can't tell if the green pepper is healthier than the red one, or that the cherry tomatoes are healthier than the large beefeaters.

How can you, as a gardener, evaluate gardening techniques to select the one that produces the healthier food? Does compost or leaf mold produce a healthier bean? Will adding kelp make food more nutritious? There is lots of marketing hype and misinformation online that might sway you one way or the other, but the reality is that you have no way to evaluate the results for nutrition. You can only do things in the garden and hope it works.

More importantly, online anecdotal information is useless unless it is backed up by lab analysis.

What Does Brix Measure?

Measuring Brix is promoted as a way to quickly measure the nutrient density of food. High Brix is equated to high nutrition, but is this really true?

Brix is a unit of measure for the total soluble solids in a sample, expressed as a percent weight. A "soluble solid" is something that is a solid in pure form but can dissolve in water. Sugar is a good example. It is solid until you mix it into water, and then it looks like a liquid. Chemists call it a soluble solid, and Brix measures these molecules in plant juice.

Brix is measured by a device called a refractometer. You take a drop of plant juice, put it on the refractometer, and take a reading. The device is simple to use, relatively inexpensive, and anyone can learn to use it in a matter of minutes.

You can measure the Brix value of any type of plant, or even part of a plant. For example, you can use Brix readings to compare different kinds of apples or carrots. Apple A might have a higher Brix reading than apple B, which means that apple A contains more dissolved solids than apple B.

A refractometer measures how light is bent as it travels through a liquid. If you look at a pencil in a glass of water, you will notice that the part of the pencil in water does not join up with the part of the pencil in the air. This is obviously an optical illusion. The water has bent the light coming from the submersed part of the pencil to make it look as if it is in a slightly different position than it really is.

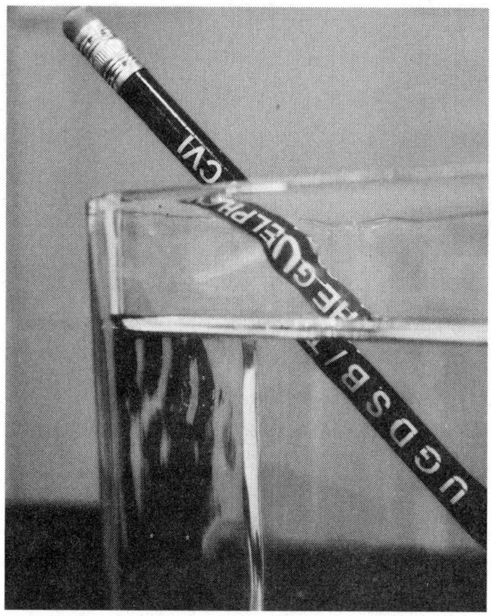

Refractive index difference between water and air distorts the pencil

The degree of bending depends on the amount of solids in the sample. If we add a small amount of chemical to pure water, we get a small amount of bending. If we add more chemicals, we get more bending. A refractometer measures the degree of light bending and indirectly measures the concentration of chemicals in the water.

A really important point here is that all chemicals bend light the same amount. A gram of compound A will have the exact same effect as a gram of compound B. Scientists have standardized on a scale, or number system, that is called Brix. We measure temperature using a Celsius or Fahrenheit scale and we measure total solids with a Brix scale.

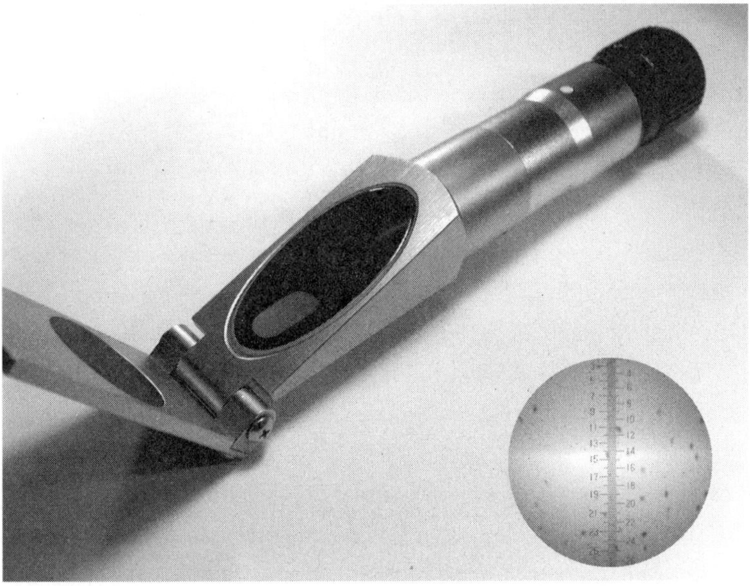

Handheld refractometer Credit: Fernando G[1]

The Brix Fallacy

Food is nutrient dense when it contains high amounts of nutrients, which means that it has a high Brix reading. In some circles, Brix is now incorrectly equated to nutrition.

The reading on a refractometer is the sum of all the solids in a sample. This includes sugar, carbohydrates, proteins, vitamins, minerals, and everything else you can think of. However, the relative impact of any one chemical on the final reading depends on the amount of that chemical in the sample.

Vitamins, for example, occur in very low concentrations, compared to, say, carbohydrates. What this means is that you could change your growing conditions to double the amount of vitamins, and you would not see a change in the Brix reading. The same is true for most minerals. Many of the chemicals that are important to our health exist in low concentrations, so changes in their concentration have little or no impact on the Brix reading.

Consider this analogy: You have a penny and a silver dollar in your pocket. You measure how much you have and come up with a reading of $1.01. If you double the amount of pennies, the reading stays about the same, at $1.02 and yet the number of pennies has increased by 100 percent.

There are two chemicals in a plant that affect Brix the most: sugar and water. Plants contain high amounts of sugar, so this chemical affects the Brix reading the most. Other carbohydrates and proteins also affect Brix because they exist in high concentrations.

A statement such as "any Brix reading above 15 means the plant is going to be high in nutrients" is nonsense. I can mix some water with sugar to make a 15 Brix solution—is that nutritious?

The chemical that has the biggest impact on Brix is water. Remember that Brix measures concentration. The solids in a sample will be diluted if the sample contains more water, producing a lower Brix reading. A grape has a much lower Brix reading compared to the same fruit once it is dried into a raisin. The total amount of solids has not changed, but the concentration of solids has.

A tomato sitting on the counter slowly loses moisture and therefore its Brix goes up over time. If you believe the Brix story, a tomato is more nutritious tomorrow than it was yesterday. The water level in a growing tomato plant also changes a lot. Stop watering your tomatoes before harvest and they will have a higher Brix reading. Water more and Brix drops.

Because Brix is mostly affected by sugar and water, it is not very useful for measuring nutrition in food.

Factors Affecting Nutrient Density

Society is discussing two key factors that affect nutrient density: soil fertility and modern cultivars. Many believe that food today is less nutritious because our soil is used up and is no longer producing nutritious crops and that modern-day cultivars have been bred to be less nutritious.

Is Soil Fertility Decreasing?

The main nutrients in food come from the soil, and if our soil is less fertile then it will affect our food. Some studies looked at the nutrient level in today's food compared to one hundred years ago and found a decrease in nutrients (more on this in the next section). This fostered the idea that soil fertility is dropping.

A new movement has developed to solve our dropping soil fertility. It wants to "remineralize" the soil by adding things like rock dust to agricultural and garden soil. The organic movement is also very big on solving these kinds of soil issues. Before we can understand the benefits of such actions, it is important to determine how big of a problem we really have. How depleted are our soils? Which nutrients are actually missing?

When we harvest fruits and vegetables, we are clearly removing some nutrients from the soil. It seems very logical that over time the nutrient level in soil will go down, but how quickly do the levels drop?

Here is an analysis I did a few years ago. Soil contains 1 to 5 percent iron—let's use an average of 2 percent, which is 400,000 mg/sq ft, in the plow layer. A carrot weighs 50 grams and contains 0.3 mg of iron. So that 1 square foot (0.09 m^2) of soil has enough iron to grow 1.3 million carrots. At an average of five per sq ft (agricultural spacing), the soil will last two hundred and fifty thousand years.

Keep in mind that the minerals come from rock, and rock is continually breaking down to release more plant available minerals, such as iron. Plants do remove some, but rocks also replace some.

Another way to look at soil mineral levels is to look at historical data for the ratio of calcium, magnesium, and potassium in plants. These macronutrients are very important for plant growth, and exist in different amounts in soils. They are also commonly added as fertilizer if levels get too low.

When the level of these three nutrients was examined over time, the ratio in plants was found to remain the same. This suggests that these nutrients are either being depleted from soil proportionally—which is very unlikely—or that they are *not* being depleted and plants are able to absorb the amounts they need. This suggests that these nutrients are not being depleted from agricultural soils.[2]

What happens when the fertility of our soil drops too low? Plants won't grow. Even if one nutrient is too low, it will stop plants from growing. If we look at agricultural yields, they are higher today than they have ever been. That simply could not happen if agricultural soil fertility was too low.

There is no doubt that agriculture removes nutrients from soil, but the amount removed for most nutrients is extremely small compared to the amount in soil. In the case of certain macronutrients, we add them back in the form of fertilizer and manure. In fact, agriculture adds more of these back to soil than the harvests remove, which can cause pollution issues. All of the science points toward the fact that soil fertility is not being depleted.

Is Food Less Nutritious Today?

In the late 1990s, several studies were done that compared the nutrient level of today's food to that of fifty years ago and they found that nutrient levels were lower today. News headlines quickly concluded that this was proof of a decline in soil fertility. Modern agriculture had used up the nutrients in our soil, and now our food supply was suffering.

If you review the studies, you quickly realize that the researchers never concluded that "our soil was depleted." They reported on the data and gave several possible explanations. It was popular press and special interest groups that cherry-picked the data that supported their cause.

Here is an example of how the press abuses the data. A popular quote for a British study is that "copper levels dropped 80%" and this is quickly extrapolated in headlines to "fruits and vegetables are 80% less nutritious." Copper was the only measured nutrient that had such a high drop. The reality is that the lower copper levels are probably due to the fact that we stopped using toxic copper pesticides during that same period of time. No one bothered to ask if the higher copper levels fifty years ago actually harmed us or if they were natural.

Here is what one of the most commonly referenced studies actually said: "As a group, the 43 foods show apparent, statistically reliable declines ($R < 1$) for 6 nutrients (protein, Ca, P, Fe, riboflavin and ascorbic acid), but no statistically reliable changes for 7 other nutrients. We suggest that any real declines are generally most easily explained by changes in cultivated varieties between 1950 and 1999, in which there may be trade-offs between yield and nutrient content."[3]

There are other issues with such historical reviews. The sampling techniques and testing procedures changed a lot during the fifty-year period, so test numbers today can't be easily compared to test results from fifty years ago. The varieties grown today have changed a lot. Due to globalization, food is now grown in different places with different soils. We know that food grown in different soils has large differences in nutritional values.[4]

There is no good scientific evidence that shows that food is less nutritious today than it was fifty years ago, with one possible exception. The varieties grown today may be slightly less nutritious, and the estimate for this drop is 10 to 15 percent. Given today's access to year-round food, at least in developed countries, this is not significant.

What Does Science Know About Growing Nutrient-Dense Food?

There have been a lot of studies that looked at nutrients in food grown in various types of soil or with different levels of fertilizer, but I found none that looked at nutrient density, probably because the term is not well defined and the cost of measuring hundreds of compounds is too high.

Allen V. Barker from the University of Massachusetts has been studying nutrients in various vegetables and found the following: Eighteen lettuce cultivars, including butterhead, romaine, and looseleaf, were tested for calcium levels and found that loose-leaf had the highest levels and romaine the lowest. Synthetic fertilizer produced higher levels of calcium than organic fertilizer. Modern cultivars produced larger heads than traditional cultivars, but the calcium concentration was the same in both groups.

In cabbage, Baker found similar results. Crop yield was greater with chemical or organic fertilizers than with compost. The mineral nutrient content (P, K, Ca, Mg, Na, Fe, Zn, Mn, Cu, Mo, and B) was not affected by the fertilization method. Modern and heirloom cultivars as a group had similar values, although there were significant differences in specific cultivars.

Similar results were found in tomatoes (P, K, Ca, Mg, Na, Fe, Zn, Mn, Cu, Mo, and B). "Differences in nutrient concentrations between modern or heirloom cultivars or among fertility treatments were small or insignificant. Differences among individual cultivars for each element were large with some cultivars having nearly twice the concentration of nutrients." On average, heirloom tomatoes produced smaller fruit than hybrids. Some believe that this means heirlooms have more concentrated nutrients, but that is not the case. The concentration of nutrients remains the same for all fruit sizes.

In greenhouse hydroponics, synthetic fertilizer increased the levels of nitrogen, potassium, magnesium, and iron in lettuce when compared to organic fertilizer, but organic fertilizer produced food with the highest phosphorus.

A review of literature on grain production shows that minerals can be increased by adding higher levels of synthetic or organic fertilizer. Fertilizing soil is most effective for increasing zinc and copper, while foliar feeding is most efficient for iron. Iodine is increased the most by adding it to irrigation water.

Five different green vegetables were analyzed for beta-carotene, vitamin C, and riboflavin content. Organically grown produce did not always result in higher vitamin levels than conventionally grown food.

Antioxidant production in tomatoes is affected by environmental conditions including temperature, light, and water, as well soil nutrients and the time of harvest, but much of the details on this are still unknown.

Our scientific knowledge on nutrient density is much more limited than the popular press would have you believe. Many types of food have not even been tested, and where they have been tested, the work has looked at only a few specific nutrients. For example, we know almost nothing about phytonutrients. Given our limited knowledge, why is there so much advice given out in gardening circles?

Here are some generalized conclusions based on the studies that have been done:

- organically grown food is not more nutritious than conventionally grown food
- heirlooms as a group are not more nutritious than hybrids, although individual cultivars might be better
- increased fertilization increases minerals in food and may increase other nutrients
- nutrient density varies significantly among cultivars, and cultivar selection seems to be more important than the way food is grown
- much of the information about nutrient density is still unknown

Is Fresh More Nutritious Than Old?

Is fresh-picked food that is eaten right away more nutritious than older food? Some water-soluble vitamins do decompose quickly and therefore are higher in fresh food. However, minerals don't decompose. Your lettuce has just as much calcium in it a month from now as it has today. Fiber decomposes very slowly, and proteins are not going to change quickly either.

Fresh is a bit better for some nutrients, but not for all of them.

Is GMO More Nutritious?

To date, the focus of creating GMO cultivars has focused on pest control, but I suspect that as we advance our genetic abilities, we will focus more on nutrition. The Golden Rice I discussed earlier is a good example of a grain that has been engineered to have higher vitamin A content. The tomato called 'Purple' has much higher antioxidants than traditional tomatoes. There is no reason why we can't produce cultivars that have higher levels of whatever nutrient society needs.

Is Home Grown More Nutritious?

As gardeners we would like to believe this to be true, but it probably isn't. The science tells us that common practices such as organic gardening do not have much effect on nutrition levels, so even though our gardens may have better soil, it might not have much effect on nutrition. It will improve yield, and one way to get more nutrients is to eat more fresh food.

It is important to point out that we know almost nothing about most of the compounds in food. It is quite possible that better backyard soil might improve some of the nutrients that have not been studied yet. We just don't know.

Online Advice

There is a lot of online advice about growing healthier food, including claims such as these:

- "organic gardening will boost nutrient density"
- "bokashi composting increases nutrient density"
- "bionutrient gardening produces nutrient-dense food"

They generally talk about nutrition or nutrient density in a very general way without ever defining the term. They then go on to claim that their favorite technique produces food with higher nutrition than other techniques, but they never provide any published scientific evidence to support their claims.

It is my strong belief that most gardening techniques are not very different from one another, nor are any of them special. If a technique adds a reasonable amount of organic matter to soil, it will improve soil. All such inputs get decomposed by microbes to essentially the same plant nutrients. Any improvement to soil health has the potential of increasing nutrition in your food. Just don't expect significant improvements.

Factors Affecting Nutrients

There are three main factors that affect the nutrient level in food: climate, soil, and genetics. As a gardener you have limited control of climate with the exception of watering. You have some control over soil and can increase the control by growing in containers or raised beds, although that is not usually necessary for good results and may actually make things worse. You have some control over genetics by selecting the best cultivars.

Climate

Climate has a significant impact on how plants grow. I live in zone 5, and we have a significant winter which means that our growing season is short. Normal large watermelons just won't mature in our short summers. Tomatoes grown in the field can only be harvested for at most three months. On the flip side, cool-growing crops such as peas and lettuce do quite well.

Warm climates also have problems. When temperatures get too high, tomato flowers won't pollinate. Apple trees need a certain number of cold days known as "chill hours," (temperature below 45°F (7°C)) in order to develop fruit buds. Cool-growing veggies like broccoli, spinach, and lettuce, as well as herbs such as cilantro and parsley, do better in cooler weather.

Your control over climate is very limited. You can control light levels by selecting the area in which you grow food. A lot of plants can be grown in part shade, but most plants grow better, produce larger plants and food with higher nutrient levels when grown in full sun. Give them as much sun as possible, especially in colder climates. In more tropical regions, some shade is beneficial to both reduce the intensity of the sun as well as keep temperatures lower. Fruiting in almost all crops is reduced or even stopped when temperatures get too high.

Water is another factor under your control. Plants grow best when they don't dry out or get too much water. Use a mulch, such as straw, to reduce fluctuations of water in soil and to reduce the need for watering. Growing in the ground requires much less watering than raised beds and containers.

It is important to understand your climate and match the food you grow to your location. You never win fighting nature.

Soil

The type of soil and the level of both organic matter and nutrients has a dramatic effect on plant growth. I have dealt with this topic in detail in my book *Soil Science for Gardeners*. As described above, it has limited effect on nutrient levels.

There is a general feeling among new gardeners that all of our soil is of poor quality and unsuitable for growing food. As a consequence, there is a huge movement toward the use of containers and raised beds and a general feeling that this is the only way to grow nutritious food. That is unfortunate because most soil is more than suitable for growing nutritious food, and growing in the ground not only reduces the cost, it also makes gardening much easier.

Soil around old homes might be contaminated with lead paint, and if you live in such a home, get the soil tested. Raised beds are a good alternative if your testing shows a high lead level. Newer-built homes tend to have soil that has been compacted too much by the heavy equipment used to build the home. This soil is difficult to dig, but it does not mean it is not suitable for a garden. Dig up the soil, add six inches of compost, and you will be on your way to a great garden. Whatever happened to a little sweat equity?

A lot of soil has lower organic matter levels than is ideal. This can be fixed by digging in more organic matter when you make the beds the first time and then practicing no-till gardening along with mulching. The soil will get better every year.

The level of nutrient levels in soil can have a significant effect on yield. The only way to know your level is to get it tested. Home kits sold by nurseries are almost useless, so get the testing done by a proper soil lab. In the US, these are inexpensive and readily available from state extension offices. In other countries, the tests tend to be expensive. An alternative is to add an inch or two of compost every year and grow stuff. If it grows properly, you probably don't have a nutrient deficiency.

Genetics

Assuming you have a reasonable climate and decent soil, the factor that affects nutrient density the most is genetics. Unfortunately, there is almost no information available comparing one cultivar to another. All you can do is grow types that produce well in your garden.

6
The Flavor of Food

Nutrition is important but let's face it, we eat because we like the taste of food. Gardeners spend hours growing a few tomatoes simply because it's the only way to get a truly great tomato taste. Taste also plays a big role in our selection of food, and manufacturers take advantage of that. It is one reason that Coke and Pepsi both exist. It's all about taste—or at least the marketing of taste.

Or is it the flavor? Are taste and flavor just different words for the same thing? Unfortunately, the use of these two terms is often incorrect.

In general conversation, we use the word taste to reflect the sensation of food in our mouth, but strictly speaking, taste only refers to the sensation that food has on taste receptors in our taste buds.

Our experience with food is much more than just taste. Take mint, for example. It does have a taste, but it also has a strong aroma (a smell), and in our mouth it creates a cooling sensation as it stimulates certain nerve endings. This overall sensation is known as the "flavor" of food and it includes the aroma, texture, and taste. Even the appearance of food affects our perception of flavor. The Flavor Extract Manufacturers Association (FEMA) describes flavor as "the entire range of sensations that we perceive when we eat a food or drink a beverage."

Flavor is largely subjective because everyone tastes and smells differently and their perceived understanding of the difference between a good and bad flavor varies a lot. For example, I find the smell of celery very strong and hate the smell. For me there is a huge difference between tomato juice that has celery in it and one that does not. My wife can't tell the difference.

The flavor of food decreases as we age for several reasons. Our sense of smell decreases with age, making taste buds more important for determining flavor. To compound the problem, the number of taste buds we have also drops after we reach fifty. As we age, we also produce less saliva, and a drier mouth is less sensitive to taste. It is quite common for older people to lament about the good old days when food tasted better. The food has not changed, but our perception of flavor has.

We evaluate flavor first by a food's appearance and color. Then we evaluate taste and aroma, and finally we experience texture. But it does not stop there; our bodies are also able to evaluate nutrition during and after digestion. We eat with our eyes. The size, shape, and color of food is what gets us to pick it up. Only then do we sense freshness, spiciness, sweetness, and all of the other sensations our mouth is capable of sensing.

Our senses do not determine flavor. We do have senses for taste, smell, sight, and touch, but flavor is created in our mind by combining all of the inputs from our senses. Flavor is in our mind, and that is one reason it is so subjective.

Appearance

Taste is very dependent on visual clues and psychological factors. For example, strawberry-based foods should be red. When such food is artificially colored green, people no longer taste strawberries. The strength of the color also impacts perceived flavor. A deep red color is perceived as having a stronger strawberry flavor than a light red color. Would you buy strawberry jam that has a nice pink color?

Our judgment of food quality, especially at the time of buying or harvesting, depends almost entirely on appearance because we can't bite into the food. Size, shape, color, structure, transparency or turbidity, dullness or gloss, and degree of damage all play a role.

A small apple has a lower quality than a large one. A red tomato is better quality than a light red one.

Aroma

Years ago in my undergrad chemistry course we were working with hydrogen cyanide and I could smell it immediately, even though the work was being done in a fume hood. No one else in my small class could detect the bitter almond smell, and they thought I was crazy. We now know that about 20 percent of the population does not have the gene that allows them to smell cyanide and those that do have the gene show different levels of sensitivity.

The aroma of food depends on its volatile compounds. These are compounds that easily turn into a gas and spread through the air, eventually landing in our noses, where we can sense them. These compounds can be very different from the ones that affect our taste buds, and humans can recognize more than ten thousand different odors.

Smells can keep us safe. We can detect potentially harmful situations such as smoke, a gas leak, and the vapors of household products such as chlorine. Bacteria growing in spoiled food also give off an odor that alerts us to the danger of eating it.

We sense odors through two different pathways. The most obvious way is directly through our nose as we breathe in. The second pathway is from our mouth as we chew food. Aromas move from our mouth into our nose as we eat. Each of these pathways are processed by different nerves going to different parts of the brain. The latter one is more important for sensing the aroma of foods and is believed to account for 80 percent of the flavor of food.

Taste

Taste is a sensation that is caused when certain molecules attach themselves to taste buds in our mouth. The four common tastes are salty, sweet, sour, and bitter. Sweet and salty are detected quickly, in less than a second, and therefore they can overpower the other tastes.

Bitter is detected more slowly, which explains why we describe some bitter food as having an aftertaste.

Umami (oo-MAA-mee) is a newly discovered fifth taste, which is described as savory and is evident in broths, cooked meats, and taco-flavored chips. Umami taste buds are responsible for sensing monosodium glutamate (MSG). There's considerable debate about the existence of a sixth taste receptor for fat, and some believe that we even have sensors for a soapy taste and a metallic taste.

Did you ever burn your tongue by eating some hot food? That burning probably damaged your taste buds, resulting in food tasting bland. Don't worry, taste buds are naturally regenerated every one to two weeks, so they will be replaced with new ones and your taste will be back to normal.

Babies and children have more taste buds than adults, which helps explain why they don't like spicy food.

Many people, called "supertasters," are hypersensitive to bitter substances. Those who perceive little or no bitter taste are nontasters. This is all controlled by genetics, and was discovered by exposing people to a bitter chemical called 6-n-propylthiouracil. About 25 percent are supertasters, 28 percent are nontasters, and the remaining 47 percent are average. The reason for this difference is that the supertasters have a lot more taste buds. They are also more sensitive to other taste sensations.

You might think that supertasters enjoy their food more than others, but unfortunately the sensitivity to bitter very often interferes with their enjoyment of salty and sweet tastes. This group of people tend to be picky eaters and dislike a lot of food. That seems to describe me quite well!

You are probably familiar with the tongue map, which identifies the location of taste receptors on different areas of the tongue. Sweet in the front, salty and sour on the sides, and bitter at the back. Chemosensory scientists (the folks who study chemical stimuli on tongues) debunked this myth a long time ago. It is a good example of how myths just won't die.

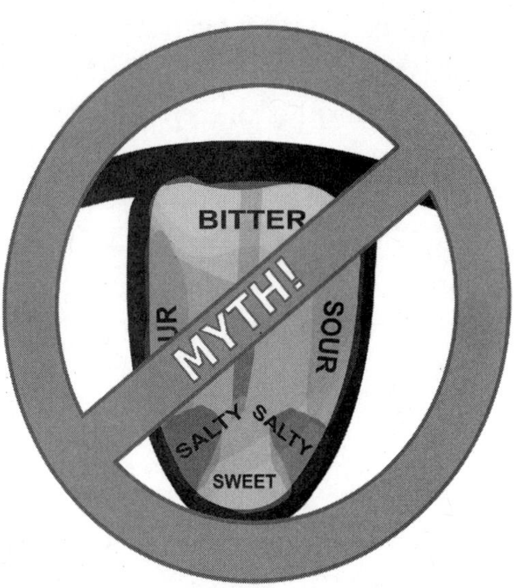

The tongue map is a myth

This myth is easy to test for yourself. Place salt on the tip of your tongue and you will taste salt.

Each type of taste bud receptor is distributed all over the tongue. Not only that, but they are found all over the mouth, including the roof of your mouth and the throat. Scientists have now determined that a specific protein is responsible for tasting sour, which is really a measure of pH. The same receptors and proteins are also found in the spinal column where presumably it is used to monitor the pH of other body fluids.

Texture

When you eat food, the tongue, teeth, and jaw apply pressure to the food, allowing you to perceive different textures. The technical term for this is "mouthfeel." Celery should be hard and crunchy, while a steak should be softer, and nobody wants soggy chips. Texture changes during cooking and storage. For example, corn is still quite solid after freezing, but broccoli gets mushy. Spy apples get soft and mushy with age. Many foods also dry out during storage, and the lack of water changes their texture. Limp lettuce that has sat on the counter for a while tastes the same as crisp lettuce from the fridge, but our perception is that one has a higher food quality than the other.

Processing and cooking food will affect texture and in turn the flavor. For example, grinding up an apple to make applesauce provides a completely different flavor. Frying foods makes them softer and also adds oils, which improve taste. Processing can also affect the appearance. Is a pureed carrot as flavorful as a whole raw carrot?

Nutrition and Flavor

What is the relationship between nutrition and flavor? Does food with high flavor also have high nutrition? Are our eating habits automatically providing us with nutritious food? These are all very good questions that science has been trying to understand for quite some time.

Other animals use taste and smell to identify nutrients essential for life. Insects are able to detect flavor compounds to differentiate between food and poison. Animals that are deficient in essential nutrients will seek them out. For example, deer and moose will find blocks of salt in winter because their bodies lack salt. Monkeys infected with parasites will go looking for specific leaves that provide relief.

A significant amount of our DNA is dedicated to creating and operating our flavor-sensing systems. Flavor is the body's way of identifying nutrition.

An interesting experiment was conducted in 1926. Dr. Davis took fifteen babies and let them eat anything they wanted from a list of thirty-four foods, including potatoes, cornmeal, barley, beef, lamb, bone jelly, carrots, turnips, haddock, peaches, and apples. There were some bizarre combinations, but at the end of the experiment all of the children were very healthy. They naturally selected food that provided them with the necessary nutrition.

The flavor compounds in tomatoes have been heavily analyzed and we now know that twenty of the most important flavor compounds are all synthesized from important nutrients. Flavor compounds are also nutritious.

Let's return to the original question. Can we use flavor to determine the nutritional level of food? To some extent we are able to do this. For example, a sweet taste comes from sugars that provide us with energy. The umami taste indicates the presence of proteins and sodium. We can sense fats in food—remember those really good doughnuts that you can't get anymore? Sour is related to important organic acids in our diet.

The problem in today's society is that a lot of food is manufactured, and companies add ingredients based on our desires and not nutrition. Potato chips are a good example. They taste better than potatoes but are not as nutritious. Many of the foods contain pleasure ingredients such as fat and sugar. We love the flavor of these, and they confuse our mind into thinking the food is good for us. Our natural animal instincts for sensing nutrition are being fooled, and we are tricked into eating the wrong food.

Food Myth: Artificial Flavors Don't Taste Right Because They Contain Too Many Chemicals

The exact opposite is true. Artificial flavors don't taste right because they contain too few chemicals. For example, artificial strawberry flavor has between five and thirty flavor and scent compounds, while real strawberries have over three hundred.

The Food and Drug Administration (FDA) defines natural flavors as substances derived from animals or plants and artificial flavors are ones that are manufactured. The actual chemicals in both types of flavors may be exactly the same, which means one is not necessarily better than the other.

It is quite possible that artificial flavors are better for you. Many of the natural chemicals have not been tested nearly as much for safety because it is just assumed that if they are natural they are safe. That may not be true.

Both natural and artificial flavors can be added to nonnutritious food to make us think it is nutritious.

Phytonutrients are nutritious, but unfortunately many of them have a bitter taste. Many have been viewed historically as plant-based toxins. Even if we breed cultivars with higher levels, people may not eat them due to their taste.

Even though we can detect a certain level of nutrition, we are not able to determine if food is nutrient dense. Remember that nutrition is the sum of thousands of nutrients and our tongue is not sensitive enough to quantify them all.

Why Does Grocery Store Produce Taste Bland?

Let's go back a hundred years or more. Many people lived and worked in rural areas where they had easy access to fresh meat and produce, at least when it was in season. Choices were very limited to whatever grew locally, but the flavor was very good.

Then things started to change. People moved to urban areas, and farms became more mechanized because they had to produce more food with a much smaller labor force. The produced food had to be shipped to towns and cities where it went through a complicated distribution system, eventually ending up in grocery stores. That fresh food was not as good by the time it made the trip.

The demand for higher quality and higher yields resulted in the development of new cultivars to solve travel problems. Now it could not only be shipped to local urban centers, but clear across the continent. We can import food from anywhere in the world and have it arrive fresh.

The breeding efforts focused on the important aspects, which were yield and transportation. In the process, flavor suffered, and today's produce is definitely lacking flavor. Along with a loss of flavor there was also a drop in nutrition, but not nearly as much as people think. It is estimated that nutrients in today's cultivars are some 10 to 15 percent lower.

It is important to remember that the drop in flavor and nutrition is balanced with access to common produce all year long. The cost of fresh food today is also much lower. A dozen oranges in 1870 sold for $11.70 (corrected for inflation).

Sweetness vs Acidity

Do low acid tomatoes taste sweeter? You would think so, but they probably don't taste sweeter. For one reason, I doubt humans can easily taste the difference between a pH of 4.1 and 4.7, which is the pH range found in tomatoes.

The second reason is that taste is a function of several compounds, and sugar (fructose and glucose) tends to mask the acid taste. When people are asked to pick the least acidic tomato in a taste test, they usually pick ones with a higher sugar content. The Super Sweet 100 cherry tomato was introduced as a "low-acid" Sweet 100 variety not because of its acidity level (it does not have low acidity), but because it tastes like a low acid tomato.

You might have noticed this sugar effect while cooking. I make a teriyaki-type stir-fry that uses both brown sugar and lemon juice. Add more lemon juice and it tastes more acidic. Add a bit more sugar and the acidic flavor is completely gone even though sugar does not change the actual pH of the sauce.

Minerals in fruit also affect taste. Both potassium and phosphate affect the acidic taste we experience. The bottom line is that we are not very good at tasting pH.

Low Acid Tomatoes

Lots of seed companies and garden blogs talk about low acid tomatoes and usually identify yellow, orange, and small fruited varieties as having low acid. Some claim that modern breeding has increased the acidity of tomatoes and that heirlooms have less acid. Others claim that there is no such thing as low acid tomatoes. The reality is somewhere between these extremes.

Gardeners talk about "low acid," but never define what they mean by the term. Nutritionists consider a tomato to be low acid if it has a pH above 4.6. Remember that low acid means a higher pH. The value of 4.6 is used because the organism *Clostridium botulinum* won't grow if the pH is below 4.6, making the food safe.

An important study from 1977 compared the pH of fifty-eight tomato cultivars grown in one Maryland location and found the pH ranged from 4.06 to 4.68. The same study also collected pH values for 356 cultivars and 212 breeding lines from research facilities across the US, covering fifty-seven different locations in twenty-three states. Both sets of data were used to reach the following conclusions.[1]

- light-colored (yellow and orange) tomato cultivars are not low in acid
- small varieties are not low in acid
- heirloom tomatoes and modern cultivars have about the same pH, although there are some heirlooms and some modern cultivars that have less acid

The range for all tomatoes growing in the same soil is between 4.1 and 4.7. This narrow range has led many authors to conclude that all tomatoes have about the same acidity, but that is an incorrect conclusion because pH is a logarithmic value. A pH of 5 does not sound much higher than 4, but since it is a log scale, it represents a tenfold decrease in acidity. That means that a tomato with a pH of 4.7 is quite a bit less acidic than one with a pH of 4.1.

If acid is causing you digestion problems or mouth cankers, you can certainly select a cultivar that is less acidic. The problem is finding such data. The above scientific references can help, but they don't contain values for newer cultivars. Seed catalogs don't provide this kind of data either and their labels of "low acidity" can't be trusted. So, lower acid tomatoes do exist—you just don't know which ones they are unless you can find their pH value in a research paper.

Factors Affecting Flavor

Almost everything we do affects flavor. The growing conditions, harvesting, storage, and the way it is preserved all affects flavor.

Growing Conditions

Every aspect of the growing environment, including soil nutrition, temperature, water availability, humidity, and amount of light affects flavor. In general, the best flavor develops when a plant is growing in ideal conditions, and that varies by plant type.

Soil fertility plays a big part. A lack of nutrients hampers plant growth, which means the plant has to prioritize how it uses the resources it does have, and survival is usually the top priority. Plants will be smaller, and contain less nutrients and fewer sugars. Plant parts such as roots and leaves may be tougher.

Table salt is sodium chloride and both sodium and chlorine are essential plant nutrients, but plants need them in small amounts. Many years ago, nitrogen fertilizer was supplied in the form of sodium nitrate, which also supplied lots of sodium. Today sodium is not used in fertilizer, and some soil now has a sodium deficiency. In that case adding table salt to soil produces better-tasting tomatoes. You have to be very careful with this because sodium is also very toxic to plants even at low levels.

Excess nutrients can also be a problem. Too much nitrogen tends to produce more green growth and fewer fruits. Such plants have thinner cell structure, are weak, and are less flavorful.

The pungency in onions is due to sulfur-containing compounds, so it should be no surprise that sulfur levels in soil play a big part in the flavor of onions. Sulfur is fairly mobile and moves through sand quickly. As a result, such soil usually has low levels of sulfur and produces milder onions. Clay holds the sulfur molecule and therefore has higher levels. It produces onions that are more pungent. Adding sulfur as fertilizer will increase pungency, and if too much is used the onions will become too pungent.

In general, soil with higher levels of clay and organic matter is more nutritious and produces better-tasting food, but such soil may not produce the best-looking food. Carrots generally taste best grown in clay soil, but they look the best when grown in sandy loam soils.

The availability of water is also important for flavor. Water is really a plant nutrient. Adequate amounts allow the plant to grow well, and deficits stunt growth. It has the same effect as low nutrient levels. Too much water can also reduce flavor. Crops such as melons, strawberries, and tomatoes taste best if they don't get too much water, especially before harvest.

Each crop has different water needs, and timing can be very important. Melons are sweeter and less mushy if they have less water near harvest time. Broccoli and kale, on the other hand, become bitter if they don't get enough water near the end of their growth cycle.

Cucumbers produce a chemical called cucurbitacin, which makes them bitter so that insects leave them alone. The amount produced in the fruit depends very much on the growing conditions and the following will help reduce bitterness:

- keep soil evenly moist—mulching can be very beneficial
- pick smaller fruit—they get bitter as they grow bigger
- cucumbers are heavy feeders, and soil with a high organic matter level will reduce bitterness
- grow in full sun

Temperature also affects bitterness. Cucumbers grow best in temperatures from 65 to 75°F (18–24°C) with a minimum temperature of 60°F (16°C) and a maximum of 90°F (32°C). High fluctuations of temperature in excess of 20°F (11°C) will cause more bitterness, as will growing at cool or hot temperatures.

Food Myth: Chemical Fertilizers and Pesticides Make Food Bitter

Research has compared the taste of tomatoes grown with organic fertilizer, ammonium-based fertilizer, and nitrate-based fertilizer. Synthetic fertilizer produced higher yields, but the taste of all three systems was the same.[3]

What about pesticides; surely they affect taste? A study of twenty-eight herbicides were tested on a variety of crops. At normal application rates, eleven reduced the flavor and two produced a slight off-taste. The rest had no effect on taste. The taste test was done by professional tasters and the effects were minimal. The researchers felt that a consumer panel is unlikely to detect a difference.[4]

You have limited control over temperature, but regular watering and mulching will keep the soil cool. In cool climates they want full sun, and in hot climates some afternoon shade will be better.

Cultivar Selection

Cultivar selection has the most important impact on flavor and is even more important than the growing conditions. Having said that, it is important to match cultivars to the growing conditions you have. There are thousands of different tomatoes, and they can all taste great if they are grown in the environment that meets their needs. Just because a cultivar has a high flavor rating in one location does not mean it is flavorful in another.

Farms who sell on a national basis have to meet the needs of the consumers' desire for uniformity. They want every apple to be the same size, color, and shape. And it has to be fresh no matter how long it has been in transit. To meet these needs, breeders have created cultivars for such a market and along the way flavor has suffered. In a more local market such as the farmer down the street, people are more tolerant of so-called imperfections and these farmers can select cultivars based on flavor. In your own backyard, you can select cultivars that grow well in your conditions and have great flavor.

The problem with selecting cultivars is that the descriptions in seed catalogs or online are not much help because you don't have full details about the environment in which they were grown. Other gardeners in your hometown are a much better resource for information.

Harvesting

Knowing when to harvest is a bit of an art form and quite honestly depends on your goal. Do you want green beans or dried beans? Are you going to make pickles or salad from your cucumbers? In each case, you would harvest at a different time.

Here is a secret for new gardeners. Start harvesting sooner than you think. If the food tastes good, keep harvesting. If it doesn't taste great, wait a bit longer. Many gardeners wait too long and end up with tough, stringy vegetables.

Remember that flavor is a combination of several factors, including taste, aroma, and texture. A very small, young carrot has great texture, but the best flavor won't develop until the plant is older and has experienced some frost. On the other hand, when the bean pod is nice and plump, showing bean seeds inside, it is already losing flavor and is getting stringy and hard to eat. Start picking radishes very early because by the time they have formed a nice-sized round ball they get woody.

There can also be a big difference between ripe fruit and ready-to-eat fruit. Nature's goal is to produce seeds, and once the seed is biologically ready to be on its own, the fruit is ripe. On the other hand, we want things to have great flavor. The green bean is tastiest just before you can see seeds forming in the pod, but it is not ripe until the seeds are large and dry.

The tomato is interesting in this regard. As the fruit ripens, it goes from a green color to a slightly red blush color. The tomato is ripe at that stage. You can test this for yourself by collecting some seeds. They will germinate, indicating that the tomato is ripe as far as the plant is concerned. We think tomatoes taste much better when they are way overripe and have a nice juicy red color.

When it comes to cucumbers, we prefer an unripe fruit. We don't want a mushy, yellow, ripe cucumber full of large seeds. We humans are a fickle bunch.

Storage

When two or more foodstuffs are stored together, one can affect the flavor and ripening process of the others. Food can transfer odors to each other. For example, apples and pears take on a disagreeable color and taste when stored with potatoes. Here are some general guidelines to prevent odor transfers:

- do not store apples and pears with celery, cabbage, carrot, potato, or onion
- do not store onion, garlic, citrus, or potato with any other type of produce

The other concern with mixed storage is with ripening. Some food produces ethylene gas, which is known as the "fruit ripening hormone." It speeds up the ripening process of certain fruits and vegetables. Placing something like a banana next to an apple will speed up the ripening process of the banana. This is discussed in more detail in chapter 7.

Slice and Dice

Slice, dice, chop, or julienne—the way food is cut also affects flavor. For example, a radish that is sliced thin provides the taste of the radish but loses most of its crunchy texture.

As food is cut, the knife damages tissue along the cut edge, which releases enzymes. These enzymes trigger chemical reactions that are responsible for much of the aroma that is given off. The liquid contents from damaged cells spill out into the sauce. Cutting smaller pieces generally adds more flavor than using large pieces. Large pieces cook more slowly so that their texture is more likely to be maintained in the final dish.

Cutting can also have a negative effect. When cut, food such as broccoli, cauliflower, and cabbage release enzymes that produce sulfur-containing compounds that are pungent. The more you cut these vegetables the stronger the flavor gets, and most people don't like it. The exact same reaction happens when onions and garlic are cut, except that their flavor is perceived as enhancing meals. It is the reason for crushing garlic cloves and sautéing onions.

I have never liked the flavor of julienne cut potatoes, but I like eating any other form of potato. There really is some science behind my madness.

7
Growing Great Food

One of the main reasons people grow their own food is nutrition. They want to eat more nutritious food, and if that is one of your goals there are steps you can take to reach that goal. Having said that, there are also limitations. The main one is that you have no way to measure the nutritional level of the food you grow. You can follow the advice I or others provide and hope that you produce nutritious food, but you never know if you actually meet that goal.

How important is it for you to grow really nutritious food? It may be better to focus on growing more food rather than really nutritious food. Let me give you an example. Let's say you grow carrots. What is more valuable to you, one carrot that has 10 percent more vitamin A or two carrots with less vitamin A? I'd go for the two carrots because the total amount of vitamins in two carrots is more than the slight increase in the one carrot. Also, you can easily count carrots and know you have grown more food, but you have no way to measure that extra 10 percent of vitamin A.

What is the difference between a carrot with high nutrient density and one with low nutrient density? There is lots of chatter about the level of nutrients, but it is important to understand that if a plant makes a carrot, that carrot has a lot of nutrients packed inside. The difference between a low nutrient one and a high nutrient one is not that great, and any carrot is better than no carrot.

In many ways, it is better for home gardeners to focus on quantity and flavor rather than nutrient density. If you grow more, you will eat more fresh fruits and vegetables and that will make you healthier. As it turns out, many of the tricks for growing more food are the same as the ones for growing more nutritious food, so you will probably reach both goals at the same time.

Focus your energy on growing food that is both tasty and easy to grow. Grow things you like. I don't care for broccoli, so I don't grow it even though it's really healthy. Grow food that is easy to grow in your soil and your climate. The focus should be on producing a lot of food and not on growing a lot of different food. You will be more successful, you will enjoy it more, and you will have more fresh food to eat.

This chapter will highlight some important tricks for growing great food, but it won't cover everything you need to know about gardening. If you are interested in more detailed information, have a look at my free online vegetable growing course on my YouTube channel called Garden Fundamentals.[1]

Selecting the Right Cultivar

Cultivar selection is one of the most important things you can do to produce great food. Each cultivar grows best in certain environmental and soil conditions, and you need to select the one that fits your conditions. The problem gardeners have is that there is almost no reliable information out there to help you with this. Social media does not work because the people giving advice don't know your conditions. Seed catalogs are of no real help either—they send the same catalog with the same information all over the country to many different environments.

The best source for information about cultivars is probably your neighbors, or the local gardening club. At least these people have tried cultivars in your conditions. The other advice I will give you is to try to grow more than one cultivar at the same time. Select the best one, and then next year grow another two cultivars, and repeat the selection process. It is really the only way to select seeds that produce well in your conditions and produce food you like to eat.

If you are a new gardener, the above paragraphs might be a bit disheartening, but it is not all gloom and doom. For some produce, the cultivar selection is not that critical. For example, lettuce. I've tried quite a few types and they all grow and produce about the same. Same with carrots; I can't tell the difference in taste and they all seem to grow for me.

If you are really new to this, I suggest you forget the seed catalogs. Go to your local nursery or hardware store and pick seeds from the rack. In most cases, they are selling cultivars that are more common and that have been good sellers for years. That means they grow well for many people. As you gain more experience, you can find better options.

What is the difference between a variety and a cultivar? These two terms are often abused by gardeners and horticulturists who tend to confuse their meaning. Varieties often occur in nature and breed true, meaning that the offspring are identical to the parents. A cultivar is selected and propagated by humans to enhance certain characteristics. They will generally not breed true from seed. Just to confuse things even more, the term cultivar means cultivated variety! Almost all types of fruits and vegetables are cultivars.

Importance of Days to Maturity

Days to maturity, or days to harvest, is a number that can be found on most annual flower and vegetable seed packets. It is a useful tool for selecting seed that will produce a larger yield, especially in colder climates. In simple terms, "days to maturity" is the time needed for the plant to produce food. Unfortunately, it is a little more complicated than that.

When do you start measuring this time period? The answer depends on how you start the seed. If the seed is usually planted straight into the garden, such as carrot seed, then the time to maturity is the time between planting and harvesting the first carrot. If the seed is usually started indoors and then planted in the garden, such as tomatoes, the time of maturity is the time from setting out seedlings to the harvest of the first tomato.

This value is useful, but it has some limitations. The above definition of the start time is still kind of vague. What if one person starts the seed directly in the ground and someone else starts them indoors? Time to maturity will be different for each person.

There is also ambiguity in the definition of harvest time. For example, you can pick carrots when they are quite small, or wait until late fall. In my zone 5 garden, that is a three-month spread. Some people let lettuce form a full head, and others pick a few leaves every week.

Location is also important. Seed companies use the same seed pack to ship over a wide range of growing zones, and plants grow faster in zone 8 than in zone 5. The days to maturity will be different in every growing zone, but the seed pack only shows one value.

Using Days to Maturity to Select Seed

The actual number is not that useful because of the abovementioned limitations. Think of them as rough guides, and use them for comparison. Radishes have a value of thirty days, and tomatoes have a value of sixty-five days. I don't expect to harvest at exactly thirty and sixty-five days, but I do know that the radishes will be ready to pick about a month before the tomatoes.

Days to Maturity for Favorite Tomatoes

Tomato variety	Days to maturity
Beefsteak	96
Early Girl	75
Sweet 100	60

Days to maturity is even more useful for selecting a cultivar. Consider the tomatoes listed in the above table. Beefsteaks will take longer to ripen than Sweet 100 no matter where you live. If you live in an area with a short growing season, it is a good idea to pick cultivars that have the smallest days to maturity value. You will be able to harvest sooner and longer before frost kills the plants.

If you live in zone 5, you also know that there is no point in planting a 140-day melon because you don't have enough growing days.

Heirlooms vs Hybrids

Heirloom seeds are reported to have several advantages over hybrids: better taste, higher nutrition, and better yields. Heirlooms also have a tradition and a story to go along with them. For example the

'Mortgage Lifter' tomato came from a man who bred his own tomato plants, eventually selling enough seedlings to pay off his mortgage, or at least that is the story that goes along with the tomato.

The term heirloom is used so much that you might think it is well defined, but it's not. Burpee, the seed company, says, "The definition is open to dispute. But the term is usually applied to fruit, flower or vegetable varieties that were being grown before World War II." A more general definition is the seed of a plant that has been carefully cultivated and passed down through many generations. *The Heirloom Gardener*—surely a source that knows the answer—says, "Some authors and heirloom aficionados say that cultivars must be at least 50 years old to be deserving of the term. Others say the cultivar must predate 1950 (a rough demarcation of the beginning of modern industrial farming practices)." The Klee Lab, University of Florida (which breeds tomatoes) says, "Anyone can call anything an heirloom if they want to. However, we loosely define an heirloom as 'old' and 'open pollinated.'"

The bottom line here is that there is no definition for heirloom seeds. There are vague sentiments about the seed being around a long time, but there is no agreement as to how long this should be. If they have to predate a specific year, 1950 for example, heirlooms will need to be at least one hundred years old in 2050. Does that make any sense?

There is also no requirement to specify quality. By most definitions, a fifty-year-old seed that produces a tiny crappy tomato is an heirloom. In theory, only the best cultivars have been saved, but in reality, much of this is done by amateurs who are free to collect and market any seed they want. That does not necessarily make it a bad process, nor does it mean that heirloom seeds are not good value for money. It does mean that almost any claim about the quality of heirlooms is going to be false, at least some of the time.

Characteristics of Heirloom Seeds

There are some common characteristics of heirloom seeds. They are not manufactured GMOs. The sweet potato is a natural GMO and you can get seed for it, which means you can have a GMO heirloom.

What Is a Hybrid?

The term hybrid is very confusing because there are at least two definitions for it.

The biological definition is that a hybrid is the resulting offspring of two animals or plants of different subspecies, breeds, varieties, species, or genera. For example, almost all the roses on the market are hybrids. If you take two different roses and cross them, you create a new hybrid. Even if you let nature do the pollination, the resulting offspring will be a hybrid. Should pollen from a rose pollinate itself, its offspring are not strictly a hybrid, but we tend to call them a hybrid anyway since their genes contain several different species.

If the pollen from a true species pollinates a different plant of the same species, it is not a hybrid and instead is called a species or a self-pollination. Seed collected from most of the perennials in the garden produce hybrids because most of them are hybrids and not species. If you cross two species, you form a "primary hybrid," and if you cross two different species in different genera, you create an "interspecific hybrid."

In the seed world, the term hybrid has come to mean something different. A hybrid seed is one where a person has moved the pollen to cross two specific cultivars of the same species. The resulting seed is also called an F1 hybrid because it is the first generation of the cross. If two F1 seedlings are crossed, they would produce an F2 hybrid.

The value of an F1 hybrid is that the breeders have very carefully selected the parents to contribute specific characteristics to the offspring. They also take steps to prevent self-pollination or accidental cross-pollination with an unwanted species. Such a cross results in superior plants that are very homogeneous.

The term open-pollinated is also used for seeds. These are seeds that nature produced using wind or pollinators. Pollen could have come from any suitable plant that is close enough. The term open-pollinated is used to distinguish these seeds from F1 hybrids. If we use the biological definition, both open-pollinated and F1 hybrids are hybrids.

What about heirlooms? They are usually open-pollinated hybrids that have been grown for a long time, but biologically they are still hybrids.

Nobody calls it that, but that is the correct label. I just checked Amazon for sweet potato seed, and most of it is incorrectly labeled as "non-GMO."

They may be grown organically, but the terms organic and heirloom are mutually exclusive. I think many beginning gardeners incorrectly think these terms are synonymous.

Heirlooms are open-pollinated, which means insects or wind selects the parents. In theory, over time these insects help line breed a variety, cementing together the best plant properties for any given location. For this to happen, pollination has to occur between parents of the same cultivar, and this presents a big problem. Since many heirlooms are produced by amateurs, there is no guarantee that there has been no cross-pollination with a different cultivar. If that happens, the resulting seed is no longer an heirloom cultivar and the fifty-year wait period for labeling it an heirloom starts over again.

Some heirlooms are handed down in families from generation to generation, but many are also produced and preserved by commercial companies.

Heirloom cultivars have been around for many years, but the documentation for them is not very good. You get seed from your granny, who got it from her granny, and so on. What evidence do we really have that the same cultivar was passed along for fifty years? How do we know it was not cross-pollinated at some point? In most cases, we don't.

There is good evidence that a number of heirlooms are available under different names, and it is fairly easy for anyone to invent a new name and call it an heirloom. I looked for a registry for official heirlooms, but couldn't find one.

Almost Heirlooms

The 'Green Zebra' tomato was introduced in 1983 by Tom Wagner. It is open-pollinated and maintains its characteristics of ripening green from generation to generation. Some call it an heirloom, and others don't because it has not been around long enough. Should age really be an important factor?

The Klee Lab, mentioned above, has tested hundreds of heirloom tomatoes, picked the best ones for flavor, and then made hybrids with them. They provide "heirloom taste without the heirloom challenges. We think they [the tomatoes] epitomize what breeders call hybrid vigor; the best of both worlds." I have tried these nonheirlooms, and they have great taste and produce well.

Brandy Boy is a new hybrid using Brandywine, a favorite heirloom. It tastes like Brandywine, has higher yields, produces an earlier crop, and is more disease resistant. Does the hybrid component really make it an inferior tomato compared to heirlooms? Should this be labeled "improved heirloom"?

There is much work being done to improve the taste of tomatoes, and we will soon have better nonheirloom tomatoes than the current heirloom ones. The same will happen with other vegetables over time.

I have grown Sugar Snap peas for many years because I have never understood the pleasure of shelling peas. Sugar Snap peas are easy to grow and very productive. I never thought it was an heirloom since everybody sells it and it's not usually marked as an heirloom. The Sugar Snap was released in 1979 by Dr. Calvin Lamborn and Dr. M. C. Parker and does not meet the fifty-year requirement, although it meets all of the other criteria.

Claims for Heirlooms

Lots of people make claims for heirlooms as a class of seeds, but this really makes no sense. How can we say all heirlooms taste better? Or that all heirlooms produce better yield? You need to consider each cultivar on its own and then decide if it has some special benefits you might want. With this understanding, let's have a look at some of the claims.

I am sure that some heirlooms taste better, but there are also many that don't. Taste is a big function of the growing environment. A particular cultivar might taste great in one location and not in another. Claiming that all heirlooms taste better is simply not true.

You can't compare heirlooms from your backyard with those

bought at the grocery store. The one is picked in an unripe state and shipped long distances. The other is left to fully ripen to maximize taste, and then, if you are like me, eaten warm right in the garden.

On a personal note, I love the hybrid cherry tomato 'Sweet 100'. I have never found another tomato that comes close in taste, including Garden Gem and Garden Treasure, from the Klee Labs, both of which are good-tasting tomatoes. Taste is very personal.

Are heirlooms more nutritious? As with taste, this is going to depend on the actual cultivar and the location in which it is grown. I would, however, argue that the Sugar Snap pea is more nutritious, at least on a per pod basis, since you eat the whole pod and not just the peas inside.

People believe that if a bee moves pollen from flower to flower, it is natural and pure. If a human moves the same pollen it is unnatural. Many heirlooms are produced by hand pollination because you can't always count on the pollinators.

Heirloom breeders select varieties that grow best in their environment. Over the years, the stronger, healthier plants are selected to produce seed. This selection process causes the cultivar to change over time to better adapt to the local environment. But you live somewhere else. If you buy someone else's seed, they are not adapted to your environment any better than hybrids would be. In fact, hybrids are usually more disease resistant in your environment. Heirlooms are only better in your environment if you buy them from a neighbor, or line breed them yourself for many years. This was made very clear to me recently when a friend brought back some heirloom Oxheart tomato seed from Italy. This is a great tomato in some places, but it never made good fruit in my garden.

Another claim is that heirlooms breed true. Clearly this is false. If it were true, they would not adapt to your environment over time. They can't genetically change to grow better and at the same time breed true. They do breed "more true" than hybrids.

Growing heirlooms preserves old strains and allows for genetic diversity. This is true, within the limits mentioned above. How important is this? Is there really value in preserving every cultivar of tomato that was ever grown? As the years go by, we will have more and more of them. Do we really need them all? Steven Tanksley, a geneticist at Cornell University, says this about tomatoes: "all that diversity of heirlooms can be accounted for by a handful of genes. There's probably no more than 10 mutant genes that create the diversity of heirlooms you see."

Heirlooms do provide a much wider range of sizes, colors, and taste compared to hybrids. Lots of people like exploring different varieties of vegetables. Historical and sentimental reasons are also important to some. Gardeners fall in love with the idea that they are part of preserving the hard work of past generations. In a recent poll I did on Facebook, this sentiment was much stronger than I had thought.

Is Organic Food Better?

The marketing effort for organic food has been very strong, and the common drivers for it is that it is grown with no chemicals, making it safer and more nutritious. Scientific testing does not support these claims.

The term organic is used in a number of different ways. Many gardeners grow food without synthetic chemicals following a number of natural techniques, and they consider their food to be organic. There are also government-led organizations that provide "organic certification," and food that is stamped certified organic has been grown following these regulations. It is important to understand that each country has their own certification standards, although the basic premise of most countries is similar.

As a gardener you are free to define organic in any way you want, but for the purposes of this discussion I will use the term organic to refer to certified organic.

It is a common belief that certified organic food is grown without chemicals, but that is a myth. The process excludes many synthetic chemicals, although the definition of what is synthetic might surprise you. Some manufactured chemicals are considered synthetic and others are not. For example, copper sulfate is considered "organic" even though it is manufactured. The most common manufacturing method uses recycled copper metal scraps and adds sulfur, which is then purified into copper sulfate.

The chemicals which are allowed in organic farming are usually less effective, resulting in their use at much higher levels than synthetic chemicals. Several organic pesticides are more toxic than similar synthetic ones that are not allowed.

Organic farming does not allow the use of GMO seed.

Taste and Nutrition

Many people, including food experts like chefs and nutritional experts, think organic food tastes better because it is grown more naturally. They believe that the organic treatment of soil transfers extra flavor into the food. Cornell University offered pairs of food to volunteers, where one was marked organic and the other was not. In reality both were identical. Most volunteers rated the organic choice as better tasting than the one labeled nonorganic. Organic marketing has promoted this "halo effect," and many consumers now believe it, but that does not make it true.[2]

There have been numerous studies that compared the taste of organic and conventional food, and most of them found no significant difference. Taste has much more to do with freshness/ripeness and cultivar selection than how it is grown.

Organic food is grown with compost and manure, which add important ingredients to soil that synthetic fertilizer just can't match. Organic gardening builds a healthy soil system full of microbes and fungi, all helping food become more nutritious—or so the story goes. In 2012, Stanford's Center for Health Policy did a very comprehensive meta-analysis of existing studies comparing organic and conventional foods. They did not find strong evidence that organic foods are more nutritious than conventional alternatives.[3]

Vitamin content was not higher. Phosphorus was significantly higher in organic food, but few people have a phosphorus deficiency in their diet, so this has little clinical value. Protein and fat contents were the same in both organic and conventional milk. A few studies did show a higher level of omega-3 fatty acids in organic food. One thing is clear. Fresh food is more nutritious than food that has sat around for a while, and this may be a bigger factor than how it is grown.

Chemical Exposure

A major concern of conventional food is the exposure to synthetic chemicals, including fertilizer, pesticides, and medication given to farm animals. There are very few studies that have actually looked at overall health and compared people eating mostly organic to those eating mostly conventional food.

A lack of chemistry knowledge leads people to think that synthetic fertilizer is somehow inferior to organic fertilizer like manure and compost, but there is no scientific basis for this. Both types of fertilizer must release nutrients in plant-available forms before plants can use them. Once in this form, both sources are identical as far as nutrients go. Neither one produces healthier food than the other.

The other important fact is that plants produce a vast number of natural pesticides—that is how they keep bugs from eating them. When you eat fruit or vegetables, 99.99 percent of the pesticides you consume are natural pesticides, and these are the same in both types of food. The remaining 0.01 percent are manufactured chemicals. It is true that conventional fruits and vegetables have a higher amount of synthetic pesticides on them, but the amounts are extremely small and well below any safety limits (see section on Chemical Toxicity).

Organically grown animals can't be given antibiotics or growth hormones, and their feed can't be exposed to pesticides, growth hormones, or synthetic fertilizer. Chickens and turkeys can be given antibiotics in the hatchery and on their first day of life. In Canada, organic dairy farmers are also permitted to give antibiotics when it's medically necessary and natural treatments don't work.

"Contrary to what you may think, the chances of you actually consuming antibiotics through animal foods is extremely low." The United States, Canada, Australia, and the European Union have strict laws that prevent contaminated meat from entering the food chain. If an animal is given an antibiotic, it must go through a drug withdrawal period before it can be sold as food. Testing by the USDA in 2010 found less than 0.8 percent of animal food products to be positive for some form of contamination, including antibiotic residue, and these were removed from the food chain.[4]

Even if there is some exposure to antibiotics, there is no evidence that they cause any health issues. The overuse of antibiotics in both animals and humans is a real and significant concern because they can lead to resistant strains of bacteria.

Buy From Local Farmers

I don't see a good reason for buying certified organic food, but there is some value in buying from local farmers—if you trust them. These local farmers do not need to be certified, they just need to farm in an organic/sustainable way. I actually think that certification produces food that is "less organic" than some conventional farms. It is certainly less "organic" than the food I grow in my backyard. But you do have to get to know the farmer and understand how they grow things so you trust them.

Be careful with local markets. It is common for the sellers at such markets to sell food they don't grow or sell imported food.[5,6]

Is local food more sustainable? The answer is very complex. I live in Ontario, and we now grow a lot of fresh food under glass, and in winter that requires the use of a lot of energy. In some cases, it is more sustainable to import the food from a warm climate that uses much less energy to grow it.

Many people don't like the idea of large multinational farms, but they generally produce food in a more sustainable way than small local growers because of the efficiencies that come from larger equipment. A recent study titled "The impact of farm size on agricultural sustainability"[7] concluded that:

- increasing farm size shows clear benefits for environmental protection

- large-scale farming is a critical path for modernizing and sustaining agriculture

Transportation by air is generally more harmful to the environment than transportation by land, but even that is changing with more efficient airplanes. Transportation by sea has a very low environmental impact compared to other means.

In some cases, local is more sustainable, and a better option. We just have to be careful not to paint everything local as better.[8]

Fresh Is Best

One of the benefits of growing your own food is the ability to harvest it at the perfect time. If you have a large garden, you can produce enough for fresh eating and canning, but if your garden is smaller, focus on producing food to eat fresh. You can always buy extra for canning.

One thing you learn very quickly is that once a fruit or vegetable is ready for harvesting, you quickly have too much to eat fresh. It is great to preserve the excess, but it is even better to design the garden so that your crop is available over a longer period of time, and there are a number of tricks you can use.

Succession planting works well. Instead of planting a 40-foot row of peas, try planting two 20-foot rows two to three weeks apart. This spreads out your harvest over a longer period of time. This method works particularly well for quick-growing crops such as lettuce and radish.

Grow cultivars with different maturity dates. Bush beans are ready for harvest before pole beans. Bush beans will produce for a longer time if you pick pods as soon as they are edible. The more you pick, the more you will get.

Some cool-growing crops stop producing in warm weather. Lettuce bolts and is finished by late spring due to the heat. The same thing happens to radish, but you can circumvent both problems. Grow some early traditional lettuce, and also plant some New Zealand spinach. This is not spinach, nor does it come from New Zealand, but it is a leafy green that grows best in the heat of summer. When your radish bolts, let it bolt. It will make seed pods not unlike peas, but they taste just like radish. Harvest the pods when they are small, and you can harvest for many months during summer.

Harvest as soon as there is something to eat. Why wait for carrots to grow to full size? You can eat both the root and the top growth of the tiny thinnings as soon as they are large enough to pull out of the ground. Instead of a big harvest in fall, harvest a few every few days all summer long.

Onion is another crop that can be harvested all season. Pick the green tops as soon as they are big enough. If you do this, the bulbs won't get very big, but that is OK. Harvest these same plants in midseason as small bulbs. Leave the tops on a few to harvest in late fall for winter storage.

Extend the Growing Season

If the goal is to grow more food, then extending the growing season will make a significant impact on your total yield. Here are some things to consider:

- Start seed indoors and use seedlings. This will provide an earlier harvest that lasts longer for many crops, especially warm-growing crops such as tomatoes.
- Cover crops with blankets or row covers early in the season and late in the season. This extra protection will allow you to plant earlier and harvest later.
- Use a cold frame to warm up the soil in early spring, which allows you to plant cool-season crops earlier. Some people even start cold-season crops such as lettuce in late winter for a really early crop.
- Use succession planting. This technique allows you to plant one crop and harvest it midseason, and immediately plant a second crop that can be harvested in fall.
- Irrigate and fertilize crops correctly so they grow at a rapid rate. Don't let the weather slow down your crop.
- Plant cultivars that have a short days to maturity value.

Harvesting Fruit at the Right Time

You can determine a cranberry's freshness by bouncing it on the floor. The higher it bounces the better they are to eat.

Fruit is the part of a plant that produces seed. It includes obvious things such as berries and fruit from fruit trees, but it also includes things such as tomatoes, peppers, beans, and cucumbers. Botanically speaking, these are all fruits because they contain seeds. The hard dry seed pods on perennials are also fruit, although we normally don't eat them.

The development of fruit is a complex process, and knowing when to harvest it is even more complicated. A simple approach that works quite well is to simply pick it, bite into it, and if it tastes good, it is ready to harvest. However, understanding the process a bit better will allow you to pick fruit at its most nutritious point.

Fruit goes through a three-step development process. After pollination, the fruits start to grow. At this stage it is usually small, green, and not very tasty. After some time, it reaches a point where it is botanically mature. The seeds have developed to a point where they no longer need the mother plant and they are able to germinate.

The third stage is the ripening process, which can take place either on the plant or after the fruit is picked, depending on the type of fruit. Some food is more palatable to us before it ripens, and other fruits taste better after ripening. Unripe apples are not very sweet, but cucumbers taste much better before they start ripening. Bananas are picked when they are quite green. The fruit is not mature yet and

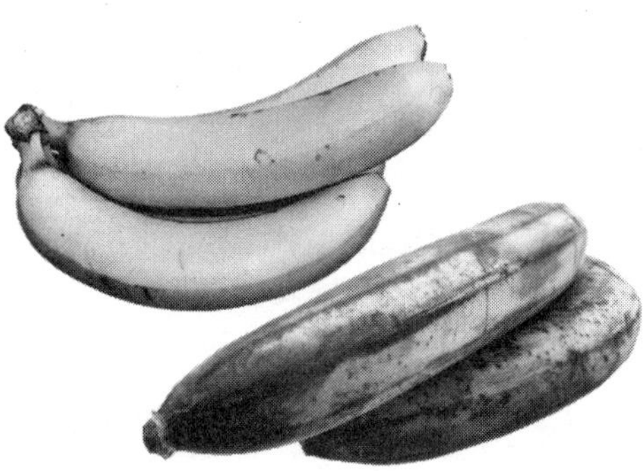

Banana ripens; some like them green, others prefer soft and sweet

seeds are just starting to develop. The same is true for snow peas and many beans. Tomatoes, on the other hand, are picked when they are well past the maturity point.

The nutritional level of the fruit increases during the maturation process, and is highest when the fruit is fully mature. Nutrition generally decreases during the ripening process, but the level of some nutrients may actually increase. During ripening, there is a major change in hormone levels with a decrease in auxin, gibberellin, and cytokinin, and an increase in abscisic acid and ethylene.

Harvesting fruit before it reaches the mature stage does two things. It limits the nutrients available, and it may prevent further ripening. Unripe fruit generally stores better and longer than ripe fruit. Once harvested, starch gets converted to sugar, making it sweeter. Texture changes, yellow and red pigments accumulate, aroma increases, acidity decreases. All of these changes occur at the same time, but each progresses at a different rate.

When should you harvest fruit? That depends on the type of fruit and your preferences. Think about bananas. Some prefer them harder and greener, and others like the sweeter, softer tissue of an almost black banana. Some fruit is normally harvested before it reaches the mature stage, including green bell pepper, cucumber, summer squash, chayote beans, okra, eggplant, and sweet corn.

Should you harvest bell peppers red or green? They are mature when they are fully grown and green. At this stage, they have a very firm texture and a slightly bitter taste, making them perfect for many culinary applications. After ripening they are red, much sweeter, and have a softer texture, making them better for fresh eating. Ripening also increases the level of beta-carotene and vitamin C. Harvest bell peppers based on your priorities and preferences. What about yellow and orange bell peppers? They are special cultivars that start out green and are fully ripe when either yellow or orange. They won't turn red.

It is best to harvest in the morning. Overnight, food regains moisture they lost during the day, making them crispier and juicier. They are also sweeter because starches that were produced during the day are converted to sugars overnight. Keep harvested food out of direct sunlight and as cool as possible, both of which will slow down degradation.

It is important to take care of the mother plant when you harvest. Gently pull off fruits so you don't damage the plant. In some cases, you will need to cut the fruit off. Peas are a good example. If you pull them off sharply, you will snap the vine, which results in no more peas being developed higher up. It is better to hold the petiole with one hand and pull the pea off with the other hand.

In many cases, frequent picking will result in more fruit being produced, resulting in a longer harvest. Plants start to shut down once they have produced mature seed, and by removing them regularly you trick the plant into growing more flowers and more fruit.

Climacteric Fruit

Fruits are classified as either climacteric or non-climacteric. Climacteric fruit continues to ripen after harvest, provided that harvesting is not done too early. This includes fruit such as peaches, plums, cantaloupe, bananas, pears, and tomatoes. After picking, they improve in flavor and get sweeter as starches are converted to sugar. Many, like peaches and plums, become soft and juicy. This group of fruit also tends to be sensitive to ethylene gas, which is discussed below.

Climacteric fruit can be left at room temperature until it is perfectly ripe, and then it can be stored in the fridge.

Non-climacteric fruit does not continue to ripen once it is harvested, so it needs to stay on the plant until it is fully ripe. This group includes berries, cherries, grapes, and citrus. That unripe orange will not get better sitting on the counter.

Ethylene Gas

You have probably heard the saying that one bad apple spoils the whole bunch. That saying is true, and caused by ethylene gas. Ethylene gas is a plant hormone that is produced by some fruit during maturation and especially during the ripening process. The hormone helps the fruit ripen itself, but since it is a gas, some of it escapes into the air around the fruit where it can also affect food that is located near the ripening fruit. A rotting apple produces excess ethylene gas, which then speeds up the ripening process of the other apples near it.

Some people will put an apple in a paper bag along with some tomatoes to help the tomatoes ripen. This works because the bag holds in the ethylene gas. It is also why you should keep apples and bananas separate, unless you like overripe bananas.

Ripening is just an aging process, and for some food we want to slow down this process. Ethylene gas speeds up the deterioration of things such as broccoli, cabbage, Brussels sprouts, and lettuce. Carrots develop a bitter flavor due to ethylene-induced production of isocoumarin. Do not store ethylene-producing produce and ethylene-sensitive produce together, and keep fully ripe fruit away from ethylene producers. You will find a handy chart for this in the next chapter under the section called Food Storage.

Food Myth: Tomatoes Ripen Best on the Vine

What is a ripe tomato? From our point of view, a ripe traditional tomato is red, juicy, and sweet, but from the plant's perspective a ripe tomato is one where the seeds are able to germinate on their own. When a fruit reaches this later stage, it is mostly green with a slight reddish blush. This is called the breaker stage. At this point in development, the plant stops sending nutrients to the fruit because it is ripe.

A tomato picked at the breaker stage and left sitting on the counter will reach a full red juicy ripeness that is just as good as if it were left on the vine. Ripening indoors also reduces the chance of animals and birds eating it before you get to it.

The fruit does not need high light to turn red either indoors or on the vine. In fact, too much sun can harm it if left on the vine, especially in warm climates.

The low temperature of the refrigerator will slow down both ripening and the production of ethylene gas. However, since the fridge is a closed container, it also concentrates the amount of the gas, making conditions worse. Modern fridges have a two-drawer system, so you can keep ethylene-producing fruit in one and ethylene-sensitive food in the other.

8
Handling and Storing Food

The moment food is harvested it starts to degrade, and that is true even if it is still ripening. Microbes on both the outside and inside are using it as their food source, and they start to digest it. This damages cell structure, opens surfaces for more infection, and results in an increase in microbe population.

There are numerous ways to slow down this process, and I've divided the discussion into three chapters. This one will deal with handling and storing food in its original condition. The next chapter looks at various ways to preserve it for long-term storage, and the following chapter deals with cooking the food for immediate consumption.

Food preservation starts right in the garden. It is best to gather food when it is cooler, either first thing in the morning or late at night. The problem with doing it in the morning is that the plants tend to be covered with dew. Spreading dew from one leaf to another is a good way to spread some fungal diseases, so it is best to avoid collecting food when leaves are wet.

Keep the food out of direct sunlight so that it stays as cool as possible. If you are collecting a lot of food on a really hot day, consider using a cooler with ice.

Washing Hands and Produce

There are three reasons to wash fruits and vegetables:

- remove dirt
- remove germs
- remove pesticides

Lots of people wash their produce, but it is also important to continually wash your hands as you handle food. Soil in the garden contains pathogens, and dirty hands carry them into the kitchen. Not washing after going to the bathroom is also a common cause of foodborne illness. Touching one type of food can transfer pathogens to another food simply because of dirty hands.

Washing hands frequently when you handle food is strongly recommended, but how well does it work? Scientists have tested this by exposing hands to contaminated ground beef followed by various washing techniques. Washing with room temperature water removed 90 percent of the germs, while using warm water removed almost 100 percent. Gloves actually collected more germs than bare hands, and washing them was less effective. The science is clear: don't wear gloves, and wash regularly with warm water.

Does soap kill germs? This is a common belief that is not true. Neither hand soap nor dish soap, which is actually a detergent, kills germs. Even the evidence for microbial soaps is weak. The reason soap works to rid your hands of microbes is that it removes some of the oils from your hands while at the same time removing the germs. When you wash your hands, the germs end up down the sink, but they are still alive.

Many human pathogens attach to food instantly and then form a biofilm that allows them to stick very tightly. The biofilm can be formed in as little as thirty seconds and once formed, the bacteria can be difficult to remove. Some can even withstand chlorinated water baths.

Some pathogens can also invade the internal parts of plant tissues through cuts and bruises. Motile bacteria, such as *Escherichia coli* and *Salmonella* are especially good at this, and once a pathogen is inside the produce, no amount of washing will remove it.

It is important to keep the wash water at the same temperature as the produce, or washing might even hide pathogens in the food. The sudden temperature drop when you wash sun-warmed tomatoes in cold water causes the gasses inside the tomato to contract, creating a hydrostatic vacuum that sucks in microorganisms. Such washing has been documented as the cause of salmonella outbreaks in both mangoes and tomatoes. The rinse water should be within 5°C (10°F) degrees of the produce.

Germs such as *Salmonella*, *E. coli*, and *Listeria* are a real concern on food. A tap water rinse removes germs as well as or better than a rinse using commercial products, soap solutions, bleach, baking soda, or vinegar solutions. The Food and Drug Administration (FDA) and Centers for Disease Control (CDC) strongly urge consumers to stick with plain running water.[1]

Here are some more tips for washing food:

- remove visible dirt from produce right away
- for the most part, don't wash until you are ready to eat or cook the food; this is especially true for berries
- don't use either vinegar or baking soda—both can affect flavor
- the wax coating on apples is edible and does not need to be removed
- never use soap, detergent, or bleach
- produce labeled as "washed," "triple washed" or "ready-to-eat" does not have to be washed again
- always wash before slicing or processing food in any way

Washing Off Pesticides

It is important to understand that 99.9 percent of the pesticides you eat are natural pesticides that are mostly found inside the food. No amount of washing, with any product, will remove them. The good news is that you don't have to remove them because they are safe to eat.

There is a wide range of manufactured pesticides, and each one has different chemical properties. Some dissolve in water and are therefore easy to wash off with plain water. Others wash off better in other solutions. For example, one study tested different solutions for washing organophosphorus pesticides (trichlorfon, dimethoate, dichlorvos, fenitrothion, and chlorpyrifos) off raw cucumber. A solution of 5 percent sodium carbonate (washing soda) worked best for two compounds, and a 5 percent sodium bicarbonate (baking soda) solution worked best for the other three. No one single solution is best for all pesticides.

DIY solutions like vinegar plus water or salt plus water can potentially react with the pesticide and produce a more toxic compound. Fruits and vegetables have pores just like your skin. Soap and other cleaning products can get trapped in the pores, and they can be just as toxic as the pesticides you are trying to remove.

For these reasons, the Food and Drug Administration (FDA) recommends washing under warm running water. It is as effective at removing pesticides as any other option including commercial washing products.

If you are still not convinced that pesticides are not an issue, there are further steps you can take to reduce your exposure:

- wash under warm running water
- scrub firm produce such as melons and potatoes with a clean brush
- discard the outer leaves of leafy produce such as lettuce and cabbage
- remove and discard the peels where possible
- heating can get rid of some pesticides

The Best Way to Wash Berries

Should you wash strawberries, raspberries, and blackberries? This is an ongoing debate with one side believing that washing berries is essential, and the other side believing that washing harms the fruit. The claim is that they absorb too much moisture, which causes them to spoil faster.

The claim that berries absorb moisture during washing is false. If you wash them and remove surface moisture, they weigh the same before and after washing.

What is the best way to wash berries? This was tested by washing in different solutions and at different temperatures. The best way to wash them is with a thirty-second dip in hot tap water. It removed the dirt as well as most of the molding spores. Fruit washed this way, dried, and stored in the fridge lasted a full week. Unwashed berries molded in three days, and the ones dipped in cold water lasted five days. Water plus baking soda made the fruit mushy. Water plus vinegar was no better than just water.

Food Myth: The Five-second Rule

The five-second rule states that if you drop food on the floor or counter, it is safe to eat provided you pick it up within five seconds. The rule is attributed to Genghis Khan, who instituted the "Khan Rule" at banquets which said that food could lie on the floor for as long as Khan allowed because food prepared for Khan was special and would not make anyone sick. Julia Child helped popularize the myth in her cooking show by routinely picking up dropped food and using it in her meals.

This rule was tested by two scientists, Dawson and Sheldon, and the results are quite instructive. First, they checked the amount of salmonella that got transferred in five, thirty, and sixty seconds. Food that stayed on the floor longer did pick up more microbes, but even at five seconds a lot of microbes are picked up. The five-second rule is clearly a myth.

Different surfaces were also tested. Tile and wood transferred about the same number of cells, with carpet transferring less. Food that was soft and sticky picked up more microbes than hard dry food.

The same work also looked at the survival rate of salmonella. Scientists spread a known amount of bacteria on tile, carpet, and wood, and counted the number of living microbes over time. The number after four hours was about the same as at the start of the experiment. The number started to drop after that for tile and wood, but for carpet the numbers were still high after eight hours. The number had dropped significantly after twenty-four hours, but the numbers were still high enough to contaminate dropped food.

All surfaces contain microbes, which attach themselves to food almost instantly. Assume all dropped food is contaminated.[2]

Food Storage

After harvesting the perfect fruit or vegetable at the peak of freshness, it's time to store it so that it maintains quality. Flavor is affected by a number of factors, including time, temperature, humidity, and light, and even the food sitting next to it has an effect.

Fresh fruits and vegetables are living tissues, and even though they are no longer attached to the mother plant, they are still biologically active. They breathe in oxygen and exhale carbon dioxide. They lose moisture to the air. Chemical reactions are taking place inside that affect both flavor and texture molecules. The ripening process continues, and eventually they begin a natural decay process (senescence). Storage conditions have a big impact on the rate of these processes. Cooler temperatures and higher humidity slow down the aging process. The tricky part is that each type of food has its own best storage condition.

Temperature

Food ages and deteriorates faster at higher temperatures, so it seems reasonable to keep it all as cold as possible. The problem with this plan is that some fruits and vegetables lose flavor faster at lower temperatures. It is a balancing act between stopping deterioration and maintaining flavor. Each crop has an ideal storage temperature, but in general, cool-season vegetables should be stored at cooler temperatures (32 to 35°F, 0 to 2°C), and warm-season crops should be stored at warmer temperatures (45 to 55°F, 7 to 13°C).

Relative Humidity

Fruits and vegetables start losing water as soon as they are harvested through a process called transpiration. The rate at which water is lost can be controlled by the method of storage, which in turn controls the relative humidity around the food. In the same way that it is hard for you to sweat on a humid day, your food also has trouble transpiring when it is placed in high humidity. This helps maintain appearance, nutritional quality, juiciness, and flavor, while at the same time reducing wilting and softening. A good example is lettuce. On the counter it gets limp fast due to loss of water. Place it in a plastic bag and the humidity in the bag keeps it turgid.

The low temperatures of refrigerators do reduce the transpiration rate, but they tend to be dry environments and that is why they include crisper drawers. These have adjustable vents that can be closed down to keep humidity in the drawer higher. It is a good place to keep vegetables that tend to lose water quickly, such as leafy greens, asparagus, broccoli, cauliflower, cucumbers, and green onions.

As mentioned above, food starts its decay process as soon as it is harvested. This is a combination of natural chemical processes inside cells and attacks from microbes. Both of these processes are more active at higher temperatures and less active at low temperatures. Placing food in a refrigerator will slow down the process significantly compared to room temperature, but there is a catch. Refrigeration can cause cold damage, called chilling injury, and it prevents further ripening.

The symptoms of chilling injury vary, and in many cases do not show themselves until the food is warmed up again. Symptoms include discoloration, surface pitting, water-soaked spots, and increased decay. Bananas are extremely chill sensitive and show signs if stored below 55°F (12.5°C) for a few days. On the other hand, honeydew melons won't show signs even after a couple of weeks at 41°F (5°C).

Each fruit and vegetable has a preferred storage temperature as outlined in the table below.

Here are some other tips for storing food:

- place each type of food in a different container to reduce the transfer of flavors and reduce the effect of ethylene gas
- use most fruits and vegetables within three days for maximum flavor and freshness
- prevent moisture loss by storing in paper bags or perforated plastic bags
- keep away from direct sunlight
- once removed from the fridge, eat them or process them right away

In general, food quality declines over time both in terms of flavor and nutrition. Freezing delays this change more than cold storage, but freezing has its own complications, which will be discussed in the next chapter.

Storage Conditions for Fruits and Vegetables[3,4,5]

	Storage temperature	Climacteric fruit	Ethylene producer	Ethylene sensitive
Apple	room	yes	yes	yes
Artichoke	fridge			
Asparagus	fridge			yes
Avocado	room/fridge	yes	yes	yes
Banana	room	yes	yes	yes
Beans—green	fridge			no
Beets	fridge			
Berries	fridge	no		no
Broccoli	fridge			yes
Brussels sprouts	fridge			
Cabbage	fridge			
Cantaloupe	room	yes	yes	yes
Carrot	fridge			
Cherry	fridge	no		no
Citrus	room	no		yes
Collard greens	fridge			yes
Corn	fridge			
Cucumber	room	no		yes
Eggplant	room	no		yes
Figs	fridge	yes		
Garlic	room			no
Grapes	fridge	no		yes
Herbs	fridge			
Honeydew	room	yes		yes
Kiwi	room/fridge	yes	yes	yes
Lemon/lime	room	no		yes
Lettuce	fridge			yes
Mango	room	yes		yes

	Storage temperature	Climacteric fruit	Ethylene producer	Ethylene sensitive
Mushrooms	fridge			
Onions	room			yes
Orange	room	no		no
Peach	room/fridge	yes	yes	yes
Pear	room/fridge	yes	yes	yes
Peas	fridge			
Peppers	room	no	yes	yes
Pineapple	room	no		
Plum	room/fridge	yes		
Potato	room			no
Radish	fridge			
Squash—summer	fridge	no		yes
Squash—winter	room	no		yes
Sweet potato	room			yes
Tomato	room	yes	yes	no
Watermelon	fridge	no		yes
Zucchini	fridge	no		

9

Preserving Food

Food is best when it reaches its peak of ripeness. Unfortunately, we like to eat every day, and not just when the food is in perfect condition. We therefore have to find ways to preserve the food.

Preservation tries to preserve freshness, flavor, and nutrition, while at the same time preventing the food from spoiling. Each technique has pros and cons, and it is important to balance not only the quality of the food, but also the convenience of storing it.

Preserving Techniques

I am using the term "preserving techniques" to include any process that is used to extend the shelf life of food. Food degrades through two main processes: microbial action and internal chemical reactions. Preserving techniques either slow down these processes or stops them entirely. Most of the common techniques are focused on controlling or eliminating microbial activity since they both degrade the quality of food and cause illness.

It is important to remember that all of the preserving techniques discussed below also affect the desirable characteristics of food. They might affect taste, texture, color, and nutrient levels, and different foods will be affected to different degrees. It is important to select the process that has the least negative effect and preserves the food item the longest. There is no perfect preservation technique for all foods. For example, zucchini does not can well, and you don't want to eat frozen cucumbers.

All of the preservation techniques discussed in this chapter use one or more of the following basic scientific principles.

Freezing Temperatures

Bacterial activity is almost completely stopped at freezing temperatures and enzyme activity is slowed down. It is important to understand that freezing does not kill all microbes, which means that both they and enzymes become active again as soon as the food is warmed.

Heat

Boiling or blanching destroys enzyme activity and kills most microbes, but not all of them. Enzymes are destroyed at about 140°F (60°C). Water boils at 212°F (100°C), which kills many microbes, but some can survive up to 248°F (120°C), which can be reached in a pressure cooker.

Added Preservatives

Microbes don't grow well in acids, and are killed in alcohol. Both environments also deactivate enzymes. Techniques such as pickling (added acids) and fermentation (produces alcohol) make use of this technique.

Other additives can also be used. For example, smoke adds formaldehyde, which has negative effects on microbes.

Osmosis

Osmosis is a process where water moves from an area of high concentration to an area of low concentration. Microbes and the cells of our food contain a fairly high concentration of water. When you surround them with a lot of sugar or salt, which contains very little water, the water from inside the cells moves into the sugar and salt, effectively drying the cells. This kills microbe cells and dries food.

This process is very effective for bacteria, but fungi, including mold and yeast, are capable of growing in high sugar or salt environments.

Exclusion of Air

Reducing the air around food starves microbes of oxygen, which they need to survive. This either kills them or forces them into a state of dormancy where they won't affect food. The seal around the food also prevents new organisms from reaching the food.

Reducing Moisture

Microbes live in water. They can survive on seemingly dry surfaces, but that is because they have a microscopic covering of wet mucus. On a microscopic level, they are surrounded by water even when sitting on your dry countertop. Removing moisture will kill them.

Methods for Preserving Food

Blanching

Blanching is a technique where food is dipped in boiling water or held over steam for a few minutes to deactivate enzymes. Each food item has a "best" blanch time, and steam blanching takes a bit longer than water blanching. University of Minnesota[1] provides an extensive list of blanching times. Blanching for too short a time is worse than overblanching because it can activate enzymes, which speeds up the deterioration of food. Overblanching can cause a loss of flavor and nutrients.

The blanching process is normally followed by freezing to prevent color changes and the development of odd tastes. Blanching does not make the food sterile.

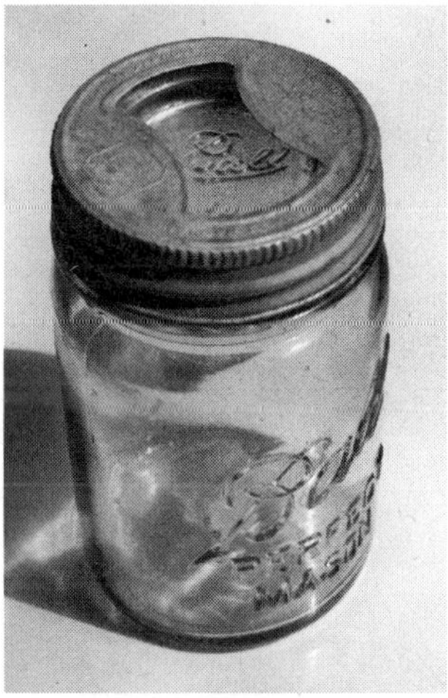

The original Mason jar with glass lid and metal cap
Credit: Jonathunder[2]

Canning

Canning was discovered by Nicholas Appert in 1809 as a way to preserve food for Napoleon's army. It wasn't until the 1850s that Louis Pasteur was able to explain that food was spoiling due to bacteria. John Mason invented the Mason jar

The Fear of Botulism

One of the main reasons people don't can foods is a fear of botulism. Food that is not preserved properly can kill you, but the risk is exaggerated provided you follow good recipes and don't cut corners. Botulism is serious but rare in developed countries.

Botulism is a poisoning that attacks the body's nerves and causes difficulty breathing, muscle paralysis, and even death. This toxin is made by a bacterium called *Clostridium botulinum*, and more rarely *Clostridium butyricum* and *Clostridium baratii*. These organisms are found naturally in many places, and they are able to make spores that allow them survive in the environment, even in extreme conditions. The spores themselves are not harmful, and can be eaten.

When spores are exposed to the right conditions, they grow and make one of the most lethal toxins known. The following conditions help them grow:

- low-oxygen or no oxygen (anaerobic) environment
- low acid (above 4.6)
- low sugar
- low salt
- a certain temperature range
- a certain amount of water

When food is canned, preserved, or fermented in a way that provides these conditions, *Clostridium* organisms grow and produce toxins. If the food is subsequently eaten, it makes people sick. When food is prepared with high acid, sugar, or salt, it prevents the spores from growing. The spores are heat resistant, but the toxin is destroyed by moderate heat (for example, at internal temperatures greater than 185 °F (85 °C) for five minutes or longer). The key to keeping food safe is to use the right conditions so that the organisms can grow.

in 1858, making the process much easier. We still use a form of his jars today.

Canning is very popular and a great way to preserve food if you have limited freezer space. The canned food can be stored in a dark dry place such as a basement, and a root cellar is ideal. There are two canning processes called water bath canning and pressure canning.

Water Bath Canning

Water bath canning is easy to do and does not require any special equipment other than some canning jars. It is also less intimidating because it does not use high pressures.

Food is added to hot, sterilized jars which are then placed into a pot of boiling water for a specified period of time. The boiling water kills off microbes, reduces the amount of air inside the jar, and helps the lid suction itself onto the jar as it cools. The preserved food is stable for months and even years.

It is important to have a rack inside the pot so that jars do not sit right on the bottom of the pot, or they might break. The lids are loosely laid on the jar so that air can escape as they are heated.

Water bath canning is safe for jams and jellies with high sugar content and for fruits and vegetables when the pH level is below 4.6. Food that can be canned using a water bath include berries, stone fruits, apples, pears, grapes, tomatoes, and pickled vegetables. Food that should not be canned this way include meat, poultry, fish, non-pickled vegetables, eggs, and dairy. The University of Minnesota [3] provides a good list of canning times for low acid foods.

Pressure Canning

Pressure canning is a similar process to water bath canning except it takes place inside a sealed pot called a pressure cooker. Why is that important? When a pressure cooker is heated, the pressure inside increases from about 15 psi to 30 psi. At this higher pressure water boils at 121°C (250°F), and is high enough to kill all microorganisms, even those that can survive a boiling at room temperature. The food inside the canning jars is then sterile. Since it kills all microbes, this canning technique can be used for almost any food.

Canning Reference Chart

Type of food	Pack type	Head space	Boiling water bath (minutes)	Pressure canner (minutes)	Dial gauge	Weighted gauge
Applesauce	hot	½ inch	25	10	6#	10#
Beans—green and wax	hot and raw	1 inch		25	11#	15#
Beets	hot	1 inch		35	11#	15#
Berries (whole)	hot	½ inch	20	8	6#	10#
Carrots	hot and raw	1 inch		30	11#	15#
Cherries (sweet or sour)	hot	½ inch	25	10	6#	10#
Corn (whole kernel)	hot and raw	1 inch		85	11#	15#
Peaches, apricots, and nectarines	hot	½ inch	30	10	6#	10#
Pears (halved)	hot	½ inch	30	10	6#	10#
Peas (fresh green)	hot and raw	1 inch		40	11#	15#
Rhubarb (stewed)	hot	½ inch	20	8	6#	10#
Soups (vegetable, dried beans/pea, meat, poultry—NO seafood)	hot	1 inch		75	11#	15#
Tomatoes (packed in juice)	hot and raw	½ inch	90	25	11#	15#
Tomato juice	hot	½ inch	45	15	11#	15#

Note: The above values are for quart jars. Values for pint jars can be found in the original source: University of Minnesota.[3]

New users have anxiety issues when they first use a pressure cooker because of a fear of explosions. Provided you follow the instruction manual for your pressure cooker, they are quite safe. They generally have a weighted top piece that prevents the pot from developing too much pressure.

Pressure canning can be used for all of the items discussed above for water bath canning as well as the items that are not suitable for water canning. In particular, it can be used for meat, poultry, root vegetables, squash, tomatoes, beans, peas, and soups. It can be used for other things, but you may not want to use it for leafy greens because they turn to mush, brassicas that become mushy, and eggs and dairy that just don't taste good.

When there is a choice between water bath canning and pressure canning, it is better to use water bath canning for taste, texture, and nutrition. Pressure canning is always safer, but is not needed for acidic food. In either case, always follow a recipe.

Pressure Cooking Myths

Myth #1: Pressure Cooking Destroys Vitamins and Minerals

Minerals are elements, such as calcium, magnesium, and iron. They can't get destroyed by any cooking or process method—that is basic chemistry. Vitamins are organic molecules that can be destroyed during processing.

The reality is that pressure cooking retains more vitamin C, B1, B2, and B6 (95 percent) than microwaving (85 percent), steaming (85 percent), or boiling (60 percent). One of the reasons for this is that any vitamins "lost" actually move into the liquid in the jar and the liquid is normally consumed.

Myth #2: The High Temperature in the Pressure Cooker Produces Carcinogens

Frying and grilling at high temperature creates carcinogens, and some have extrapolated this to conclude that the high temperature in pressure cookers will do the same. That is simply not true.

Temperature is not the only condition that produces carcinogens. In a frying pan, the oil and lack of moisture contribute to its creation, while in a pressure cooker the food is bathed in water, an environment that is not conducive to creating carcinogens.

Myth #3: Pressure Cooking Sterilizes Food

Pressure cooking does sterilize food, but as soon as it is exposed to air, it becomes contaminated again. Once you open a jar that has been pressure treated, it is no longer sterile, nor are leftovers.

Dehydrating

This is a simple process. Take some food, cut it into bite sized pieces, and dry it. Once it is completely dry, it lacks the water that is needed for microbes to grow. The dried plant cells also prevent enzymes from being active, preserving flavor and nutrition for the most part. However, some change in taste, color, and texture is normal, and dried fruit may become sweeter. Changes in texture are reversed to some extent when the food is rehydrated.

Dehydration can be done in the sun, in an oven, or in a specially designed electric dehydrator. The secret is that the process needs to happen slowly and at a fairly low temperature. Slight warming speeds up drying, but it should not get too hot.

A condition called case hardening happens when the temperature is too high. The outside of the food pieces dry quicker than the inside, resulting in a hard outer shell that traps moisture inside and prevents proper drying. It is always a good idea to check a few pieces by cutting them open and making sure they are fully dry.

Best Dehydration Temperatures

Food item	Dehydration temperature
Herbs	95°F (35°C)
Most vegetables	125°F (52°C)
Beans and lentils	125°F (52°C)
Fruit	135°F (57°C)
Grains	145°F (63°C)
Precooked meats	145°F (63°C)
Meat, seafood	160°F (71°C)
Poultry	165°F (74°C)

If faster drying is required, it is better to slice food into thinner pieces rather than increase the temperature. Food can be blanched before drying to stop enzymatic activity and limit changes in flavor. The foods that lend themselves to dehydration include berries, fruits, vegetables, legumes (beans and lentils), grains, pasta, low-fat meats, seafood, and fat-free sauces. The following foods do not dehydrate well: fatty foods, avocados, dairy products, and eggs.

I've done a lot of hiking and canoeing trips, and I never leave home without some dried banana chips, pineapple chunks, and cranberries. They make the perfect snack on the trail.

Freeze Drying

Freeze drying, or lyophilization, is a process in which water is removed from food after it is frozen. This is done by applying a vacuum to convert the ice into water vapor, which is removed. The quick removal of water retains much of the food's original flavor and nutrition even after rehydration.

This is a two-step process. The food is first frozen to a low temperature. The lower the temperature, the more efficient the next step is. The food is then placed in a vacuum machine that draws air out using a pump. Once the food is completely dry, it can be stored at room temperature in plastic bags or jars. It is a good idea to add a moisture-absorbing pack or to keep them in the fridge, which tends to be drier. Vacuum packing is a common method for longer-term storage.

Freeze drying does not kill bacteria. Scientists even freeze dry bacteria to preserve them for future studies. Provided the food is kept mostly free of bacteria before freezing and the drying process is complete, the food is safe to eat. How do you tell if the drying is complete? The resulting food should be "crisp" and easily breakable. Food that has high sugar levels will not be as crispy, but they should not be sticky.

Both nutrition and taste are well maintained with this method. Freeze dried food rehydrates more fully than dehydrated ones, making them taste better, and the nutritional levels from this method are better than most other preservation methods. Studies have shown the method is very good at preserving anthocyanins, flavonoids, and vitamin C.

Here are some tips for freeze drying:

- Cut fruits and vegetables into evenly sized portions so they freeze and dry at equal rates. The size should match the size you want for final eating or cooking of the item.
- Lay food in one even layer before placing in the freeze dryer.

- Prefreeze in a regular freezer. Once frozen, the food can be stored frozen for a while until you are ready to dry it.
- Foods that have a high sugar content or a thick membrane (such as blueberries) take longer to dry. Cutting thick-membraned fruit makes it easier for the water to escape.

Drying Seeds

This process can be used for things such as beans, peas, sunflower, squash, and various smaller seeds used as spices. It is important that these seeds are grown to maturity on the plant. In some cases, like beans, they should be very dry before picking. The seeds rattle inside the pods when ready. Sunflowers should also be allowed to remain on the plant until they easily separate from the flower.

The harvested seed is then shelled, cleaned, and dried some more. This can be done at room temperature provided the humidity is not too high. You can also dry them in an oven at 100°F (38°C) for several hours.

Once completely dry, they can be stored in jars or gauze bags. If you do store them in jars, check on them from time to time to see if any condensation has formed inside the jar. If it has, the seeds were not dry enough before storing. Dry them again. The advantage of gauze bags is that they can continue to dry even after storage.

Rehydrating (Refreshing)

Before using dehydrated products, it is a good idea to "refresh" them by soaking or cooking them in water. This should only be done right before you are ready to use them. The refreshing times on the table can be shortened by using warm or even hot water.

Fermentation

Fermentation is a process where microbes change the properties of food by converting organic molecules such as carbohydrates and sugars into antimicrobial metabolites (organic acids and alcohol). These compounds prevent the growth of pathogens. There are two

Refreshing Dehydrated Food

	Amount of water per 1 cup dried food (in cups)	Minimum soaking time (in hours)
Beans, green snap	2½	1
Beets	2¾	1½
Carrots	2¼	1
Cabbage	3	1
Corn	2¼	½
Okra	3	½
Onions	2	¾
Peas, green	2½	½
Squash	1¾	1
Spinach	1	½
Sweet potatoes	1½	½
Turnip greens, other greens	1	¾
Apples	1½	½
Pears	1¾	1
Peaches	2	1¼

Credit: Barbara Willenberg, *How to Use Dehydrated Foods*[4]

general forms of fermentation: lactic acid fermentation and alcoholic fermentation.

Lactic acid fermentation is carried out mostly by bacteria, the common being lactic acid bacteria or LAB for short. They convert the sugar lactose into energy and lactic acid, which lowers pH and keeps microbes from growing. This type of fermentation is used to preserve pickles, sauerkraut, cheese, and yogurt.

In alcoholic fermentation, microbes convert sugars such as glucose into energy, alcohol, and CO_2. This is carried out by yeast, fungi, and some bacteria, producing leavened bread, wine, and beer.

Alcohol is toxic to most microbes, so why would yeast produce it? It turns out that many yeast species are more tolerant of alcohol than other types of organisms. By producing alcohol, they are killing off the competition.

Fermentation is used to both preserve food and make food more palatable. Fermented vegetables and cheese can last much longer than the fresh ingredients. In the case of olives, fermentation makes bad-tasting food edible. In recent years, various fermented foods such as yogurt and kombucha are seen as providing healthy probiotics to help balance gut bacteria.

The process is fairly simple and requires little or no special equipment, making it ideal for home use. Fermentation can be used on many fruits and vegetables, and even dairy products. It is not suitable for meat, seafood, potatoes (unless you are making vodka), or leafy greens.

Health Benefits of Fermentation

Fermentation provides several potential health benefits:

- They contain potential probiotic microbes such as LAB. These organisms are protected from stomach acids by the food and they do survive long enough to enter the gut. The amount and type depends very much on the type of food being fermented.
- The microbes produce a variety of compounds during fermentation that may provide health benefits. For example, LAB produces bioactive peptides (pieces of protein) that may benefit our immune and cardiovascular systems.
- Microbes convert various compounds into biologically active metabolites.
- Fermentation can also reduce toxins found in the food. For example, it reduces the phytic acid concentration from soybeans.

There is no doubt that fermented food provides nutritional value in our diet while also preserving it. However, the science supporting claims such as the above list are still very preliminary, and many sources exaggerate the benefits.

Most testing to date has used in vitro studies where tests are done in the lab. One of the few randomized controlled trials for gastrointestinal effects were for kefir, sauerkraut, natto, and sourdough bread. No such tests have been performed for kombucha, miso, kimchi, or tempeh. The most widely investigated fermented food is kefir, with evidence from at least one study suggesting beneficial effects in both lactose malabsorption and *Helicobacter pylori* eradication. Although in vitro studies are positive, there is very limited clinical evidence for the effectiveness of most fermented foods on gastrointestinal health and disease.[5]

There is much talk about our gut microbiome, but the reality is that we know very little about it. We do know that it changes with time and that most of us seem to have a unique microbiome. The knowledge we have about food's effect on our gut is quite limited, and most claims are speculative. For example, claims that fermented food "balances" our microbiome have very little basis because we don't really know what a balanced gut microbiome looks like and we don't know how the food affects it, except in some very general ways.

It is quite possible that the microbes in fermented food are beneficial to our gut. If that is true, then it is important to consume such food that contains living microbes. Cheese, for example, is fermented, but it usually does not contain living organisms except for the fuzzy fungi on some cheeses. Yogurt may or may not contain living organisms, depending on how it was made.

Making fermented food is fairly risk free provided you follow established recipes. It can be contaminated during or after fermentation, in which case there is some risk of food poisoning.

Some fermented foods should also be ingested in limited amounts. For example, you should not drink more than twelve ounces of kombucha per day. Drinking too much can lead to headaches, nausea, diarrhea, rash, and even stomach cramps. Kombucha can also contain vinegar nematodes, which are small, worm-like animals. They won't harm you, but they might be unpleasant to drink.

Bread

You probably don't think of bread as a fermented food, but it is. The fermentation process produces carbon dioxide, which forms the bubbles in baked goods. Have you ever smelled rising yeast dough?

Fermented Foods and Drinks

Kefir	Kefir grains (yeast and bacteria) are added to milk to produce a thick, tangy beverage that tastes similar to yogurt. It is believed to aid in digestion and reduce gut inflammation. Bacteria break down lactose in the milk so kefir has less lactose than milk.
Kimchi	A popular Korean side dish made from fermented cabbage, radish, and other vegetables. It is easy to make and can be added to many dishes.
Kombucha	Fermented green or black tea that's tart, flavorful, and carbonated. It is made by combining tea with SCOBY (symbiotic culture of bacteria and yeast). The yeast converts sugars and tannins into ethanol, which the bacteria then turn into acids. It is now available in grocery stores, although commercial products may contain high sugar levels. If it is made at home it is important not to over ferment it or it will become too acidic. Normal kombucha has a pH of 3.5.
Miso	Made by fermenting soybeans, salt, and koji, a type of fungus. It is the main ingredient in miso soup, a traditional Japanese breakfast. It has been associated with lower risks of cancer and stroke, although the high salt content may cause other health issues such as stomach cancer.
Natto	Made from fermented soybeans, it has a strong taste and slimy texture. It contains a high level of fiber, protein, and vitamin K. Natto is a staple probiotic food in traditional Japanese cuisine. It contains an enzyme called nattokinase that is used to treat blood clots and lower blood pressure, but the amount in natto is not enough to have much of an effect.
Sauerkraut	A popular side dish made by fermenting shredded cabbage with lactic acid bacteria. It has high fiber and vitamins C and K. It also contains the antioxidants lutein and zeaxanthin, which are claimed to benefit eye health. It can be added to many dishes but is a natural side dish to sausage.
Tempeh	Fermented soybeans that have been pressed into cakes forming a high-protein substitute. It can be baked, steamed, or sautéed before being added to other dishes. It has a high nutrient level and may contain antioxidants. It is a good option for vegetarians.
Yogurt	Milk that has been fermented with lactic acid bacteria (LAB). The bacteria convert the sugar lactose into lactic acid, which gives it a unique texture and tart flavor. It is high in protein, calcium, potassium, phosphorus, riboflavin, and vitamin B12. A number of health benefits have been claimed for yogurt. In order to see these benefits, it is important to eat yogurt with living probiotics. Some commercial products have been pasteurized to kill the probiotics.

It smells kind of boozy due to the alcohol that is produced. Unfortunately, much of this evaporates during baking.

Beer

Beer has been made for thousands of years, and it is believed that the original yeast used was *S. cerevisiae*, the same yeast used to make bread. It is still the most popular yeast used to make ale.

This ale yeast is a top-fermenting yeast, which means that it likes to float to the top of the beer as it creates alcohol and carbonation. It performs best between 50 and 70°F (10 and 21°C) and is used to make a wide range of beers, including witbiers, stouts, ambers, and IPAs.

A different species, *Saccharomyces pastorianus*, is also used to make beer, but it is a bottom-fermenting yeast that works best between 48 and 58°F (9 and 14°C). It was discovered by Bavarian brewers about two hundred years ago and is now responsible for the majority of beer produced worldwide. This lager yeast is used to make Pilsners, lagers, bocks, and many others.

Belgian beers have a very unique taste that comes in part from using many unusual yeasts. These yeasts tend to produce a lot of phenols, esters, and clove flavors, giving the beer an earthy flavor, which sounds terrible, but believe me, it tastes great.

How important is the type of yeast when it comes to flavor? Very important. If you take the same ingredients and change only the yeast, you will produce a different tasting beer.

Wine

Wine is made from yeast-fermented fruit, usually grapes. As sugar is used up by the yeast, the concentration of alcohol increases. At some point the concentration gets too high and kills the yeast. If this happens before all of the sugar is consumed, the wine will turn out to be too sweet.

Some yeast can tolerate a higher concentration of alcohol than others, which makes the selection of yeast very important.

Fruit can be processed using the natural yeast found on it, and this process is called natural or spontaneous fermentation, which results in flavor complexity. If done right, it produces a higher quality of wine, but it is not without risk. The process could stop prematurely, or not start properly. Off-flavors can develop with the wrong kind of yeast. Because of these issues, most winemakers inoculate the must (fruit juice) with a culture of active dry wine yeast.

Champagne and sparkling wines are made using champagne yeast. These are special strains of *S. cerevisiae* that produce more CO_2, tolerate higher alcohol levels, and produce a clearer-looking product with a mild taste. This yeast is also a good selection for homemade wine since it's not as fussy about temperature and nutrient levels, making it easier to use.

How important is yeast selection for flavor? Experts attribute about 50 percent of the flavor to the yeast with the remaining flavor coming from the fruit itself. A common approach to making commercial wine is to use three different yeasts in three fermenters and then blending the final product to get the perfect taste.

Freezing

Freezing can be used to preserve most produce for a fairly long period of time; however, it comes with a cost. The process of freezing alters the texture, and both high and low temperatures can cause a decrease in quality known as "freezer injury." Whether injury occurs depends on the commodity. In some cases a single freezing will cause damage, and in other cases even repeated freeze-thaw cycles cause minimal damage.

During the freezing process, water turns to ice and the sharp ice crystals cut cell membranes. This damage appears as a loss of rigidity, softening, and water soaking. The effect is reduced if the food is warmed up slowly and if it is not handled during the thawing process. These changes are also less noticeable in high-starch vegetables, such as peas, corn, and lima beans.

A slow freeze causes the water outside of cells to freeze first. This draws water out of cells through osmosis, causing cell walls to rupture, changing its texture and making it softer once it is defrosted. A quick freeze results in less water movement and less cell damage.

These suggestions will help preserve the flavor of produce:

- freeze at peak ripeness
- use small, made-for-freezer packaging (smaller sizes freeze faster)
- seal the package with as little air as possible
- freeze as quickly as possible
- eat the oldest frozen food first

Freezer burn is characterized by dry tough layers on the outside of the food. This is caused by a loss of moistures and is really not a burn. The ice crystals near the surface of the food sublime and turn into water vapor. This water vapor escapes through the packaging, leaving behind dry cells. Airtight, thicker, walled containers reduce freezer burn. Food with freezer burn is perfectly safe to eat, although the quality may not be as good.

The water in frozen food is unavailable to bacteria. Many do survive the process, but they can't reproduce and their biological activity is almost stopped.

You can freeze any fruits and vegetables, but a few just don't taste good after freezing, including cucumber, zucchini, celery, endive, lettuce, and radish.

Added salt and sugar will lower the freezing point. In fact, all the compounds in food will lower its freezing point. For example, desserts freeze between 29.5 and 26.6°F (–1.4 to –3.0°C) depending on the concentration of sugar. The higher the sugar concentration, the lower the freezing temperature. Salt in our food is usually in low concentrations compared to sugar, so its effect on freezing is limited. Home freezers operate at about 0°F (–18°C), a temperature that is low enough to freeze all of this food.

Frozen Food Myths

Myth #1: Freezing Kills Bacteria and Viruses

This is simply not true. Freezing inactivates microbes so they stop growing, but they are still alive and will start growing as temperatures increase. Viruses can even survive freeze drying.

Myth #2: Frozen Foods Aren't as Healthy as Fresh Foods

Food nutrition starts dropping once food is ripe. Freezing slows down this process and is therefore healthier than food that has been refrigerated for five days. Freezing is one of the best ways to preserve the nutrition of food.[6]

Myth #3: Frozen Food Has No Expiration Date

From a safety point of view, frozen food does not have an expiration date provided it is stored continuously at 0°F (–18°C) or below, but from a quality point of view, it does. Water slowly moves out of frozen food, drying it over time, changing its flavor.

Storing Frozen Food

Suggested storage time	Frozen food item
1–2 months	bacon, sausage, hot dogs, lunch meats, pizza, chicken nuggets
2–3 months	vegetables, soups, and stews containing meat
3–4 months	ground beef, lamb, pork
9 months	chicken , turkey
4–12 months	beef

Credit: "Cold Food Storage Chart," Food Safety.gov.[7]

Myth #4: Frozen Foods Are High in Sodium

Salt is not added to frozen fruits, vegetables, or meats. Frozen premade dinners may have higher salt levels, which should be specified on the label.

Myth #5: Frozen Food Can Be Thawed on the Counter

Freezing does not kill microbes and as soon as food thaws, these microbes start to grow. It is better to thaw food in the fridge, or quickly in cold water. Once food is thawed, keep it in the fridge until you are ready to cook it.

Myth #6: Refreezing Thawed Food Is Unsafe

Food that has been thawed at room temperature for more than two hours should not be refrozen because of the buildup of microbes. However, it is perfectly safe to refreeze food that has been thawed in the refrigerator or that has been cooked after thawing. Flavor may be affected by refreezing.

Oil Packing

Oil seems like a good way to preserve vegetables because it keeps air out, preserving the color and texture of food. The lack of air should prevent microbes from growing, but that is not the case for all microbes. Some molds and pathogens such as *Clostridium botulinum*, the organism which causes botulism, grow quite well in oil.

In the 1980s there was a serious outbreak of botulism in Canada and the United States caused by chopped garlic stored in oil. Authorities reacted by banning the sale of some garlic-in-oil products.

Provided the pH of the oil is below 4.6, the pathogens won't grow and that is why most recipes call for the addition of vinegar (acetic acid) or citric acid to the oil. Even with this extra step, oil-preserved vegetables should be stored in the fridge and used within six months.

A common belief is that some herbs, spices, and garlic in particular have antimicrobial properties. This is true, but the effects are not very strong and they will not keep all microbes from growing in stored food.

Pasteurization

Pasteurization is used for milk, fruit juices, and beer. The resulting product is not sterile, but the bacterial count is quite low and pathogens are normally destroyed. Pasteurization makes milk safe to drink, but if left warm, bacteria grow and form lactic acid, which sours the milk. The process also denatures some enzymes, which is the main reason for pasteurizing fruit juices.

Pasteurizing milk can be done at home by using a very clean double boiler and heating the milk to 150°F (63°C) for at least thirty minutes or 162°F (72°C) for at least fifteen seconds. Cool the milk quickly in an ice bath, and refrigerate right away. Done properly, it will keep for two weeks.[8]

Juices and cider can be pasteurized in a similar way. Use a double boiler and heat to 158°F (70°C) for at least one minute while stirring frequently. Transfer to sterile jars while still hot.

Pickling

Pickling is a food preservation method that uses vinegar, water, salt, and sometimes sugar. The food is immersed in a low pH liquid and then canned. The acidic condition prevents the growth of pathogens and gives food a unique taste while allowing it to be stored for a long time. In fact, most pickles need to be aged before they reach their peak of deliciousness.

Pickled food can taste similar to fermented food, so what is the difference between the two methods? Pickling is done by putting food into an acidic brine solution, which gives the food an acidic taste, whereas fermented food tastes acidic due to the fermenting process. In general, pickling is the less healthy of the two options.

The Difference Between Fermenting and Pickling

	Fermenting	Pickling
Is vinegar used	no	yes
Does it need to be stored in the fridge	yes	yes if cold packed
Does it contain probiotics	yes	no
Is it easy to make	no	yes

There are two basic kinds of pickles: the traditional canned pickles and the quick pickles, also called refrigerator pickles. The latter are really easy to make. Fill a jar with sliced vegetables and some spices. Mix 1 cup of water, 1 cup of vinegar, 1 tsp salt and 1 tsp sugar. Bring the liquid to a boil and almost fill the jar. Store them in the refrigerator and start eating after forty-eight hours. They will keep for about two months. It doesn't get any easier than that.

Both pickling processes can be used for just about any fruit or vegetable and even hard boiled eggs—one of my favorites. I like to use the leftover juice from canned pickles as the liquid to make pickled eggs. You might need to add a bit more vinegar to help the taste.

Salt is an important ingredient and it should be canning or pickling salt, which does not have the anti-caking material that is added to table salt. Do not reduce the salt level found in recipes and don't use sodium-reduced salt.

Food items tend to get soft during the picking process. To combat this, many recipes add a firming agent, usually alum, which is a double sulfate salt of aluminum with the formula $XAl(SO_4)$, where X is either potassium or ammonium. Alum is considered to be a safe food additive by several agencies including the US Food and Drug Administration (FDA), European Food Safety Authority (EFSA), UK Food Standards Agency, as well as the Joint FAO/WHO Expert Committee on Food Additives (JECFA). There is some concern that aluminum in higher amounts can be a health issue, and many commercial products have reduced the use of alum. As a result, many store-bought pickles are not as crisp as they used to be.

Health Benefits

Is pickled food good for you? Overall, the answer is a definite yes. Most of the nutrition that was in the original fresh food is still in the food. The vinegar is not harmful to you. Acetic acid is part of your biochemistry and is naturally found in your body. Drinking pickle juice has become a trend because of touted benefits related to muscle cramps, weight loss, and diabetes. There is some scientific support for these claims, and it is the vinegar that provides the benefits.

It is important to understand the terminology. Unfortunately, American English uses "pickles" and "pickle juice" to include both fermented and vinegar pickles, and that confuses discussions about health benefits. In the UK, "pickle" refers to Indian pickle condiments. The abovementioned benefits are attributed to pickle juice made from added vinegar.

There are also lots of other claims for the probiotics in "pickle juice," but only fermented products contain probiotics. Pickles made with added vinegar do not contain probiotics, and therefore won't do much for adding bacteria to your gut.

Pickles can increase your intake of antioxidants that are naturally found in all fruits and vegetables. These compounds are sensitive to heat, and cooking destroys them. Pickling without heat preserves them.

The high salt content is a drawback for most people, but it can be a benefit for people who need higher sodium levels. It is also a good reason for not drinking pickle juice.

Salting

Salt is an effective way to preserve food because it reduces the available water, and without water microbes can't survive. Preserving food solely with salt is no longer a common practice, but it was very important historically. Salted meat and fish were very common before the invention of refrigeration, and salted lemons are still popular in many regions of the globe. Smoked salmon also goes through a salting stage.

Salt still remains an important ingredient in many of today's preservation techniques.

Vacuum Sealing

Vacuum sealing can be applied to a wide range of food items, both fresh and cooked. It will extend the shelf life of food from two to five times as long, depending on the type of food. Once sealed, food can be kept at room temperature, in the fridge, or in the freezer.

Some harmful bacteria grow better at low oxygen levels, so vacuum packing makes it easier for these to grow. In most cases, vacuum packing needs to be combined with another preservation technique, such as cold storage, to make the food safe. Dry food, such as crackers and nuts, can be stored at room temperature.

The process is fairly simple. Place the food item in a plastic bag, remove the air, and seal the bag to prevent air from getting back in. The reduced oxygen level prevents microbial growth and reduces natural changes in flavor due to oxidation. The reduced air also prevents freezer burn.

Most food can be vacuum sealed, but a few are not recommended including soft cheese, bananas, mushrooms, whole apples, raw onions and garlic, cabbage, leafy greens, and cooked vegetables.

Irradiation

Irradiation is a commercial technique where high energy radiation is applied to food for twenty to thirty minutes to kill microbes and insects. Food does not become radioactive, nor does radiation leave any residues.

International standards have been established by experts from many countries, making the process extremely safe and highly regulated. Respected international organizations, such as the American Medical Association, Centers for Disease Control, and the World Health Organization, endorse the safety of irradiated foods.

The radioactive cobalt that is used for irradiation is recycled material from material used to sterilize medical equipment, and all of the material produced in North America could be stored in a space equal to an office desk.

There is some loss in nutrition, but the loss is equivalent to leaving food sitting for a couple of days. There is no change in taste, but irradiated food is much safer to eat.

10

Cooking Food

This chapter will discuss cooking methods that are used to prepare food, with a focus on immediate consumption. It will answer the question, how does cooking affect flavor, nutrition, and microbes? Cooking is a process that produces safe, edible food by combining ingredients with heat (in most cases). It is a way of making food fit for human consumption.

Why Do We Cook Food?

Cooking food has several benefits:

- improves digestibility
- improves flavor (taste, texture, and appearance)
- warms the food
- preserves nutrition
- reduces toxicity
- reduces the number of microbes

Warming food does not add a lot of health benefits, but it does make many foods more pleasurable to eat. The other benefits of cooking are more important for our health.

Digestibility

We eat to satisfy our hunger, but from a biological point of view, the main reason we eat is to gain nutrients. For that to happen, we have to be able to digest the food we eat, and much of our food is not digestible if it is eaten raw. Cooking starts the digestion process and makes it easier for our bodies to extract the nutrients from it.

For example, our digestive system is not very good at dealing with complex starches and fiber. Cooking can start breaking down these polysaccharides so that an enzyme called amylase, which is produced in our digestive system, can break them down into glucose.

Flavor

Flavor is a combination of taste, texture, and appearance. It helps us enjoy our food, which in turn helps us eat the food we need. Cooking has a huge effect on flavor and our ability to enjoy food. The humble potato can be turned into a golden, crispy French fry that changes our whole gastronomic experience.

Safety

Raw food tends to harbor food poisoning bacteria that will make us ill. Cooking at a temperature over 158°F (70°C) is a great way to kill these organisms. It is important to understand that killing these organisms does not get rid of any toxins they have already produced. This is why food that has been left at room temperature may still not be safe to eat even after thorough cooking.

Bacteria are killed more easily in acidic conditions, and therefore high-acid foods such as tomatoes and some fruit need less treatment time. Protein, fats, and sugar protect bacteria from heat because they slow down the transfer of wet heat, so food that is high in these needs a longer treatment.

As cooking temperatures rise, there is an exponential increase in bacterial deaths. So a high temp, short duration is usually best to preserve food quality while at the same time keeping it safe.

Washing and cooking food can remove heavy metals to some extent. Rice is one grain that can have higher levels of arsenic, and washing it before cooking can reduce the level by 10 percent. There are two ways to cook rice. You can cook it with the right amount of water so that when you are finished there is no water left. This method retains the arsenic level. The second way to make rice is to boil it in an excess amount of water (six cups water for each cup of rice). When the rice is done, the remaining water is discarded, reducing the arsenic by another 50 percent.[1]

How Does Cooking Affect Flavor?

Heating causes both chemical and physical changes. The effect depends on the type of food and the method of cooking. Some of these changes impact food in a positive way, while other changes are negative. Cooking is a balancing act between preparing good-tasting food and producing healthy food.

Osmosis Affects Taste

Cooking fruits, such as apples and strawberries, in water affects their taste. Through a process known as osmosis, water moves into the fruit and sugars leave. The fruit becomes plumper, especially if the fruit had been previously dried, such as raisins. They are less sweet, although the cooking liquid gets sweeter. Pectins inside the fruit become soluble and tend to move out of the fruit. Cellulose is softened, fruit becomes tender, and loses its turgor.

When the same fruit is cooked in a sugar solution, the effect is quite different. Fruit won't take on water, and its shape and turgor will be maintained. Sugar moves into the fruit, making it sweeter. This is the preferred way of cooking many berries.

In general, the taste of food becomes milder when cooked in water as some taste molecules leave the food and water is absorbed by the food.

Caramelization

Caramelization produces the characteristic color and taste of many foods such as dark beer, coffee, and roasted peanuts. The reaction takes place when starchy food is exposed to high, dry heat. The sucrose in the food melts and undergoes a process of caramelization where it first decomposes into glucose and fructose, which are then converted into hundreds of compounds. These compounds add a unique color and taste to food.

This process happens between 230°F and 356°F (110°C and 180°C). One of the most important compounds produced is diacetyl, which has a strong butterscotch taste. Also produced are furans and maltol, which add a sweet burnt taste. The final flavor depends on the type of carbohydrate found in the food being cooked and the temperature used. In general, higher temperatures produce a taste that is less sweet and more bitter. For example, caramelizing table sugar at 230°F (110°C) produces a light golden brown color along with an intense sweet taste. Processing at 410°F (210°C) produces a dark brown color and a bitter burnt taste.

Any food that contains a high level of carbohydrates (e.g., onions, apples, bananas, leeks, and carrots) can undergo caramelization if they are subjected to roasting, grilling, baking, or frying.

Maillard Reaction

The Maillard reaction is a complex chemical change that occurs in many foods including toast, meat, and baked goods. It is a chemical reaction between amino acids and sugars that happens with heat. It produces hundreds of different taste and color compounds, which vary based both on the food ingredients and the heating method.

Much of the savory taste of cooked meats can be attributed to the Maillard reaction and the production of sulfur containing compounds.

This reaction can be produced by frying, baking, grilling, and roasting.

Loss of Pigmentation

There are three classes of pigments, including chlorophyll (green), carotenoids (yellow and red), and flavonoids (white, red, blue, and purple).

Chlorophyll is responsible for photosynthesis, and can be found in most fruits and vegetables. It is fat soluble and therefore can be lost to fat during cooking. Cooking initially starves chlorophyll of oxygen, and food becomes deep green. As cooking progresses, the pigment is degraded by acids in the food and turns a gray-green color. Even more cooking turns it a yellowish color.

Carotenoid pigments are found in many fruits and some vegetables such as peppers and carrots. It is also fat soluble and is lost in cooking fat. Cooking causes oxidation of the pigments and results in paler-looking food.

Flavonoids are found in most fruits and vegetables, and are water soluble. They leach into water during soaking and boiling. Cooking methods such as stir-frying are better at preserving these pigments.

Protein Denaturation

Proteins are large molecules with a distinct three-dimensional structure. Heat causes denaturation, which is an unraveling of the molecules. Such proteins lose their function, and it usually causes changes in texture. Heating egg whites causes the clear runny material to solidify and change to a solid white as the proteins lose their structure.

Denaturation of proteins can also produce softer textures. The protein collagen gives meat its tough chewy nature. When it is heated, the protein denatures and reacts with water to form gelatin, which makes the meat softer and easier to eat.

Since this denaturation happens as a result of heat, any form of cooking will have similar results. Acids will also denature proteins.

Polysaccharide Degradation

Starch is a form of polysaccharide, which are long chains of sugar molecules. When cooked in water they form a three-dimensional structure somewhat like a fishnet. This structure traps water molecules and thickens the liquid. This is what happens when you use starch to thicken a stew.

Any food that contains a lot of starch, such as potatoes, wheat, rice, and pasta, undergo a similar reaction when heated in water.

Many plants contain cellulose and pectin, which are also polysaccharides. These molecules give the plant structure and rigidity.

Cooking breaks these molecules down into sugars, resulting in softer food. This is why most vegetables become softer when they are boiled, fried, grilled, roasted, or baked.

How Does Cooking Affect Nutrition?

There are two types of vitamins: water-soluble and fat-soluble. As the name implies, each group dissolves in a different type of liquid. Water-soluble vitamins tend to be found in food that has a high water content such as fruits and vegetables. Fat-soluble vitamins are found in higher amounts in foods such as meat, dairy products, vegetable oils, and fish.

The solubility of vitamins affects how easily they are leached out of food during cooking. Water-soluble vitamins are more easily lost in boiling, while frying and grilling loses more fat-soluble vitamins.

Both types of vitamins are also very sensitive to heat, and are degraded by both high heat and long cooking times. Stir-frying and steaming help preserve them.

Minerals are not affected by heat, but they can leach out of food when it is boiled in water since most minerals are water-soluble.

Are Raw Vegetables Healthier than Cooked?

Many people think raw vegetables are more nutritious than cooked, but that is usually not the case. A lot of the nutrients in raw vegetables are hard to extract by our digestive system and are simply lost. Cooking starts the digestive process for us, releasing more nutrients for our bodies to use.

The amount of some nutrients, such as vitamins, are reduced during cooking, but other compounds, such as antioxidants, are increased. For example, cooked carrots, spinach, mushrooms, asparagus, cabbage, and peppers supply more antioxidants, such as carotenoids and ferulic acid, to the body when cooked.

Spinach and Swiss chard both contain high levels of calcium, but they also have higher levels of oxalic acid which binds to the calcium, making it unavailable in our digestive system. Heating releases the calcium for easier absorption by our intestines.

Eating cruciferous vegetables, such as cabbage, broccoli, and Brussels sprouts, releases an enzyme called myrosinase, which produces anti-cancer compounds called isothiocyanates. Since heating destroys this enzyme you get more isothiocyanates if you eat these vegetables raw. On the other hand, indole is formed when you cook cruciferous vegetables, and indole helps kill precancerous cells before they turn malignant.

There is no simple answer to the debate between raw or cooked. It may depend on the nutrients you need in your diet. There is no point preserving vitamin C by eating raw if your diet already contains excessive amounts, which is common in many developed countries. In that case, it might be better to cook the food to increase the level of antioxidants.

Comparing the healthfulness of raw and cooked food is complicated and there is still much we do not know. In most cases, the best advice is to prepare the food in such a way that you'll eat more of the good things and don't get too hung up on the cooking method.

Cooking Creates Undesirable Compounds

Cooking changes the chemistry of food, and the process can create both desirable compounds as well as dangerous ones. The compounds listed below have been shown to cause cancer when large amounts are fed to lab animals. However, it is much more difficult for science to show a link between the normal dose of these compounds consumed by humans and cancer.

In the case of HCA and PAH, population studies have not shown a link between cancer and cooked meats. Based on all of the evidence, the International Agency for Research on Cancer (IARC) has classified red meat to be "probably carcinogenic to humans." The method of cooking can affect the amount of these chemicals you consume.

Nitrates

Are nitrates bad for you? You have probably heard that nitrates in processed meats cause cancer. The real story is much more complex. For example, beets have a natural high level of nitrates and their juice has been credited with lowering blood pressure and enhancing exercise performance. The average European diet gets 5 percent of their consumed nitrates from meat and 80 percent from vegetables.

The nitrates discussed here are identical to the nitrates in fertilizer, and plants naturally absorb them from soil. Leafy greens, such as spinach, celery, and carrots, also have high levels. This same chemical is used to preserve meats like ham, bacon, salami and some cheeses, to prevent the growth of bacteria.

A normal diet will provide you with about 1.5 mg of nitrates per day. That may go as high as 300 mg after a large spinach salad or a shot of beet juice. This level can start to affect blood pressure and levels of 2,000 mg can be acutely toxic, but are unlikely by eating food. There are cases of this level after drinking fertilizer water.

Nitrates on their own are quite safe to eat. Unfortunately, nitrates can be converted into other nitrate compounds that are carcinogenic. The bacteria in our mouth converts nitrate to nitrite, another nutrient found in soil, and nitrite reacts with amino acids in protein in the strongly acidic environment of the stomach to form nitrosamines.

Nitrosamines are also formed in food during cooking, especially at high heat or over open flames. Such cooking also forms other harmful compounds such as PAHs (polycyclic aromatic hydrocarbons) and HCAs (heterocyclic amines).

Nitrosamines

Nitrosamine compounds are considered potential carcinogens, and they exist at low levels in food and water. They are found in cured meats, fish, beer, cocoa, vegetables, cereals, milk, and in fermented or pickled foods. In short, they are everywhere.

It is claimed that they are found in the highest concentrations in smoked, grilled, and fried food, but this seems to be an exaggeration. Some studies have shown that the levels are even higher when food is boiled.[2]

It is probably safe to say that nitrosamines are not healthy in our diet, but the science on exactly how harmful they are is still not clear. Cooking does increase the amount in food, but other potentially harmful compounds are also increased and it is quite possible that it is these other compounds that are the real problem. There seems to be a wide gap between what science actually knows and what is believed in popular culture.

Polycyclic Aromatic Hydrocarbons (PAHs)

Polycyclic aromatic hydrocarbons (PAHs) are both natural and by-products of incomplete combustion of materials such as coal, oil, gas, and wood. They are also found in food when cooked over these materials both due to contamination and the actual formation of PAHs during cooking at high temperatures.

PAHs include a wide range of chemicals, including benzopyrene, benzoanthracene, benzofluoranthene and chrysene, which have varying degrees of carcinogenicity. These compounds are also found in other cooked food. The European Food Safety Authority (EFSA) has established a Maximum Residue Limit of 2 ppb in edible oils. Testing has found average levels of 0.2 ppb in baked goods, 0.3 ppb in oil, and 1.2 ppb in roasted vegetables, although roasted vegetables were found with values as high as 9 ppb.[3]

These compounds are common in food, but levels are much higher when the food is cooked at high heat in a grilling process.

Heterocyclic Amines (HCAs)

Heterocyclic amines (HCAs) are another group of carcinogenic and mutagenic chemicals that are formed from cooking beef, pork, fowl, and fish at high temperatures. More of these compounds are formed when meat is overcooked or blackened.

Acrylamide

Cooking high carbohydrate food, such as potatoes and cereal-grain-based foods, using high temperature techniques such as frying, roasting, and baking can produce acrylamide. The natural sugars and the amino acid asparagine undergo a chemical reaction that produces acrylamide. This compound is considered to be a potential carcinogen by the Food and Drug Administration (FDA), who recommends limiting it in diets.

There are things you can do to limit exposure to acrylamide and still enjoy potatoes:

- use wet cooking methods such as boiling and mashing
- store potatoes at room temperature before cooking
- cook for shorter periods of time; aim for light brown instead of dark brown
- limit the consumption of fries and potato chips

Food Myth: Cooking with Aluminum Is Bad for Your Health

Rumors about high levels of aluminum being involved with Alzheimer's disease have circulated for many years. Aluminum is a very common element and is found in water, soil, and the food we eat. It is also used as additives in products such as antiperspirants, cosmetics, and aspirin. This level of exposure does not seem to be an issue.

Cooking with aluminum foil or aluminum cookware does add aluminum to food both as soluble ions and as solid flakes of metal, but our bodies are able to handle this.

Aluminum toxicity does exist and over time can be dangerous to your brain, bones, and muscles. Such exposure usually happens in industries such as mining and the production of aluminum metals.

According to the Center for Disease Control (CDC), aluminum in cooking is not a concern. The aluminum in our food leaves the body quickly in feces or urine. Acidic foods pick up more aluminum from foil or pots, especially at high temperature, but these do not add enough aluminum to our diet to be concerned about. Cooking with aluminum is safe.

Food That Needs Cooking

Sprouts are considered to be very healthy, but they are also a perfect place for bacteria to grow. They are grown in warm, moist conditions that are perfect for bacterial growth. Wash and cook them before eating them.

Many of our foods can be eaten both raw and cooked, and the choice is a matter of preference. There are, however, a few foods that should not be eaten raw.

Dried beans contain high levels of phytohaemagglutinin, a type of lectin, that can cause red blood cells to clump together and cause nausea, vomiting, stomach upset, and diarrhea. Active lectins can interfere with the absorption of minerals, especially calcium, iron, phosphorus, and zinc. Dried beans, especially red kidney beans, should be cooked before eating. It is common to soak beans overnight, but there is little advantage to doing this if they are going to be cooked in liquid anyway. There may be some advantage to soaking if you fry the beans.

Green beans also contain lectins, and concentrations vary quite a bit depending on cultivar. Eating a few green beans raw won't affect most people, but it is a good idea to cook them first.

Raw potatoes contain both solanine and lectins, both of which can cause gastric issues, so it is better to cook them. Sweet potatoes are hard to digest, and only release more nutrients and starches after being cooked. They and yams don't contain solanine because they are not members of the nightshade family.

Uncooked eggs are not safe to eat unless they are pasteurized and even then it is not a good idea to eat them raw because they can still be contaminated with bacteria. The risk of salmonella poisoning is quite low, but since cooked eggs are just as nutritious as raw eggs, why take the chance?

Cyanide is naturally occurring in raw cassava. Properly soaking and cooking cassava will make these compounds harmless, but the water used should be discarded. You also find cyanide in apple seeds, which should not be eaten.

Lima beans contain a compound called linamarin, which releases cyanide when it is consumed. Cooking destroys the enzyme that produces the cyanide. The cyanide level in commercially grown lima beans in the United States is fairly low and must be less than 200 mg/kg. Imported beans can be much higher. Our bodies can handle a certain amount of cyanide provided we have a sufficient level of protein in our diet.

All parts of the elderberry including stems, leaves, twigs, roots, bark, and fruit contain a group of compounds called cyanogenic glycosides, which can induce cyanide poisoning if ingested. It is not harmful to touch the plant, but it should never be consumed. When it comes to berries, they should not be consumed either raw or dried. Once cooked they are safe to eat.

Fiddleheads are the young unfurled growth of ostrich ferns and are considered a delicacy. When eaten raw or improperly cooked, they cause symptoms resembling food poisoning. The cause has not been researched, but it is believed to be a natural toxin. When cooked thoroughly, for ten to fifteen minutes until tender, they are safe to eat. Don't reuse the water that was used to boil them. Sprouts from other types of ferns should not be eaten. Some are toxic even if cooked, and others are carcinogenic.

How Cooking Affects Solanine Levels

Plants in the nightshade family, including potato, eggplant, tomatoes, ground cherries, and peppers, contain a toxic compound called solanine. The common advice is to cook these vegetables to reduce the solanine level, but cooking has a minimal effect. For example, boiling potatoes reduces solanine by 1–3 percent, microwaving by 15 percent, and deep frying (410°F (210°C)) causes a loss of 40 percent. Freeze drying and dehydrating potatoes has a minimal effect.

The majority of solanine in potatoes is found in the skin, so peeling can reduce the amount between 30 and 80 percent. Fried potato peels can have values as high as 1.5 mg/g, while the upper safety limit is 0.2 mg/g.

Food Myth: Rhubarb Leaves Are Toxic

Gardeners will eat rhubarb stalks, but they won't eat the leaves because "they are toxic." I have even seen concern about adding the leaves to the compost pile because they might make other vegetables toxic. The chemical that is causing all of this concern is oxalic acid, which is toxic to humans.

This concern for toxic rhubarb started during World War II, when food was in short supply and people started eating whatever they could find, including rhubarb leaves. Several people died from them, or at least that is a story floating around. The truth is that people probably ate the leaves, but there is no documented case of poisoning.

I really encourage people to think logically about gardening information, and this is a perfect example. The rhubarb "stalk" is actually the leaf petiole—it is part of the leaf. Why would a plant develop a lot of oxalic acid in part of the leaf and not in the other part of the leaf? This never made sense to me.

A little research revealed some interesting facts. The amount of oxalic acid in rhubarb leaves and rhubarb stalks is about the same, as one would expect from basic plant biology. More interesting is the fact that the level of oxalic acid in some common foods is even higher than rhubarb leaves:

- carrot–0.5 g/100 g
- chives–1.48 g/100 g
- parsley–1.70 g/100 g
- radish–0.5 g/100 g
- rhubarb leaves–0.5 g/100 g
- rhubarb stalks–0.5 g/100 g
- spinach–0.97 g/100 g

Clearly, rhubarb leaves are not toxic, but they don't taste very good, at least not raw.[4]

You can get a rough idea of the solanine level in potatoes by tasting a raw piece. Solanine is bitter. An immediate burning sensation indicates a value over the 0.2 mg/g safe level.

Cooking Myths

Myth #1: More Bleach Is Better

It is believed that since bleach kills bacteria, using larger amounts works even better. The reality is that a small amount is as effective as a large amount. To effectively clean kitchen surfaces, use one teaspoon per quart of water.

Myth #2: Cooked Food Has No Bacteria

Cooking can kill bacteria, but it does not sterilize the food. As the food cools, the remaining bacteria start to grow. Bacteria from the air are also added if the food is not fully covered.

Myth #3: Marinades Are Acidic and Kill Bacteria

Not all marinades are acidic, and bacteria can grow even in the acidic ones. Always marinate food in the fridge to reduce microbe growth.

Cooking Methods

There are many methods for cooking food. This section will compare the pros and cons of each method with an emphasis on preserving food quality. Some cooking methods are a healthier option, but flavor and convenience are also important considerations. The best cooking method is probably the one that gets you to eat more fruits and vegetables.

Cooking methods can be broadly categorized into dry heat and moist heat. Dry heat cooking uses an oven or open flame without added liquid, and includes roasting and baking. These methods use higher temperatures and give a nice brown coloration to tender meat, cookies, buns, and cakes. Cooking in oil is also considered a dry cooking method. Moist heat cooking exposes food to a liquid, such as water, steam, vegetable stock, or wine. These methods include boiling, steaming, and poaching, and tend to be used for tougher meat, lentils, pasta, rice, and vegetables.

Baking/Roasting

Baking and roasting are essentially the same thing. The term baking is more commonly used for making cookies, bread, and pizza, while the term roasting is used for cooking meats. Both methods are done using dry high heat in some type of oven. Baking is usually done at a lower temperature.

Both methods result in a nice brown coloration due to caramelization and Maillard reaction. The formation of unhealthy compounds can be minimized by cooking to a light brown as opposed to a very dark color.

Pros:

- enhances flavor by affecting both taste and color
- spices are easily applied before or during cooking
- even cooking throughout the food

Cons:

- starchy food such as potatoes produces acrylamide
- slow method of cooking
- tends to dry out food

Boiling/Poaching/Simmering

Given today's appliances, a wide selection of pots and their versatility, this is probably the most common method of cooking. Boiling, poaching, and simmering are all moist heating methods. The difference between the three methods depends on the temperature of the liquid. Boiling is done at the boiling point of the liquid (water, bouillon, stock, milk) while simmering is done at a slightly lower temperature and poaching is done at an even lower temperature than simmering.

A lower temperature cooks food slower and tends to preserve nutrients more. A lower temperature is also more delicate, and is ideal for things like eggs and fish. Simmering is usually done by first reaching a boiling point, and then reducing the temperature for the duration of the cooking time. Slowing down the cooking process also allows food to absorb more of the liquid and is commonly used for pasta and rice.

All three methods result in nutrients moving from the food into the liquid, and many people try to recapture these by using the water in other dishes such as soups and stews, or using it to water plants. This may recapture nutrients, but it can also recapture harmful compounds, such as arsenic from rice. The reality is that the amount of "good" nutrients in this water is very small and it is not worth saving, unless you can use it right away.

There is a lot of talk about the loss of vitamin C to the water, but people forget that boiling degrades vitamin C. So the vegetable water won't contain any vitamin C.

Pros:

- fast cooking method
- easy and foolproof
- lower temperatures produce fewer harmful compounds

Cons:

- some loss of nutrients to the water
- boiled food has less taste

Food Myth: Vegetable Water Is Good for Plants

All kinds of chemicals will leach from food into boiling water, and some of those even color the water. The general perception is that such water is "full of nutrients" and a good way to use it is to fertilize plants. The reality is that this water contains very few nutrients. It won't harm plants, but it does not add much value for the plant.

Pasta water is also used and it contains mostly starch and maybe some salt. The starch is a food source for microbes, while the salt can be toxic to both microbes and plants.

Rice water is claimed to be good for reducing diarrhea, making skin softer, preventing dandruff, and watering plants. The water will help plants but the rest of it is mostly starch, which won't do much for plants.

Frying/Stir-frying/Sautéeing

All three methods use oil and are considered to be a dry form of heating because no water is used. Sautéeing and stir-frying are essentially the same. They use a higher temperature, a small amount of oil, and the pieces of food are normally cut small, resulting in fast cooking. Frying, or pan-frying, is done at lower temperature with a bit more oil and the food is left as large pieces, resulting in a slower cooking process. When food is totally immersed in hot oil, it is called deep-frying.

Quick cooking helps preserve nutrients, and less oil is healthier. The key is to get the pan hot enough before adding the food. Low heat results in food absorbing too much oil, making it taste greasy. The invention of the nonstick pan has almost eliminated the need for any oil.

Why is oil cooking hotter than cooking with water? Water boils at 212°F (100°C) and once it reaches that temperature, it won't get any hotter. Oil, on the other hand, cooks at around 350°F (177°C). It is the chemistry of the liquids that determine the heat.

The type of oil also affects the cooking process both in terms of flavor and its smoke point. The smoke point is the temperature at which the oil starts to produce smoke. Ideally, you keep the temperature below the smoke point since the chemicals in smoke are neither good for eating nor breathing. Vegetable oil has a high smoke point, which means it only produces smoke at high temperatures. Medium smoke oils include olive oil and butter, which smoke at a medium heat. Nut oils such as sesame oil smoke at even lower temperatures.

Pros:

- quick method
- simple; a lot of ingredients can be cooked together
- adds taste and an attractive appearance

Cons:

- requires close attention to prevent scorching or burning
- foods can taste oily
- oil adds calories to food

Smoke Point for Cooking Oils

Almond oil		221°C	430°F
Butter		177°C	350°F
Coconut oil	refined, dry	204°C	400°F
Corn oil		230–238°C	446–460°F
Corn oil	unrefined	178°C	352°F
Lard		190°C	374°F
Olive oil	refined	199–243°C	390–470°F
Olive oil	virgin	210°C	410°F
Olive oil	extra virgin	190°C	374°F
Palm oil	fractionated	235°C	455°F
Peanut oil	refined	232°C	450°F
Peanut oil	unrefined	160°C	320°F
Pecan oil		243°C	470°F
Rapeseed oil (Canola)	refined	204°C	400°F
Rapeseed oil (Canola)	unrefined	107°C	225°F
Sesame oil	unrefined	177°C	350°F
Sesame oil	semirefined	232°C	450°F
Soybean oil		234°C	453°F
Sunflower oil	semirefined	232°C	450°F
Sunflower oil		227°C	441°F
Vegetable oil blend	refined	220°C	428°F

Source: wikipedia https://en.wikipedia.org/wiki/Template:Smoke_point_of_cooking_oils

Grilling/Broiling/Barbecuing

These techniques use dry heat and add flavor through the processes of caramelizing and the Maillard reaction. Grilling and barbecuing are usually done over an open flame, while broiling is done with heat in an oven. Barbecuing can also be done over burning charcoal or wood, which adds a smoky taste.

High temperature grilling produces carcinogenic compounds such as HCAs (heterocyclic amines) and PAHs as fat and protein drippings fall on hot surfaces. Grill marks might look good, but they are not healthy to eat. You can reduce the amount of carcinogens by turning meat regularly and using tongs so less meat juice falls on the coals. Keep the grill clean.

Cooking With Oil Can Be Toxic

What happens to oil when it is heated? It undergoes a process called oxidation, which can produce harmful by-products including free radicals. Higher temperatures result in more oxidation and more harmful chemicals.

As the oil gets hotter, it reaches a point where smoke is also produced. This smoke contains a lot of these compounds. To document this process, scientists measure the smoke point, the temperature at which smoke starts to be produced. Many people recommend using oil with a low smoke point because they are safer, but that is only partially true.

Oil that is kept below the smoke point still produces harmful chemicals through the process of oxidation. If they are not released in the smoke, they remain in the oil and are ingested when you eat the cooked oil. Science is now paying more attention to these chemicals.

It is now clear that the smoke point is not related to the amount of oxidation. Take olive oil for example. Many people caution against using it for cooking because it has a low smoke point. The fear is that olive oil will produce more hazardous chemicals than oil with a higher smoke point. The reality is that many of the oils with a higher smoke point produce more oxidation at low temperatures. Olive oil, on the other hand, is very stable at lower temperatures and resists oxidation better than most other oils. This characteristic is called "oxidative stability." So although it smokes sooner, it actually produces fewer harmful chemicals.

The health concern for heated oil needs to take this oxidation into account. Olive oil seems to be one of the safest oils to use—just keep it below the smoke point.

There is another aspect to the concern over heating oil. The oxidation process adds chemicals to the oil each time it is heated. Reheating oil results in an accumulation of these chemicals, which makes reheated oil the least healthy option. Studies have shown that reheated oil in restaurants can accumulate quite high levels of chemicals and many of these contribute to diseases such as cardiovascular disease and cancer.

Oil is safe to use for cooking. Keep the temperature lower, and don't reuse heated oil.

Pro:

- produces a nice taste, especially on meats

Con:

- requires close attention to prevent scorching or burning

Blanching

Blanching is done by dipping food into boiling water for five seconds to two minutes. It is not really a cooking method as much as it is a way of preparing food for another process such as freezing. It can be used to heat some fruits and vegetables before serving.

It can also be used to make skin easier to peel. For example, blanched fruit is much easier to peel. It does not kill most microbes, and has minimal effect on taste, texture, or nutrition. It can stop enzymatic activity, which prevents further loss of quality.

Pros:

- can make peeling easier
- improves digestibility
- may improve the color of some food

Con:

- extra work

Microwave

Microwaves are electromagnetic waves that transfer energy to water, causing it to heat up. The hot water in turn cooks the food. Compared to other processes, it is fast and therefore may cause less damage to food.

This process maintains a high level of antioxidants in many vegetables and even increases it in some, such as eggplant, corn, peppers, and Swiss chard. Vitamins that are sensitive to heat are still degraded, but since the cooking time is short, the amount lost is less than with other, slower cooking methods.

Heating plastic in the microwave can release bisphenol A (BPA) and phthalates from various plastics. Microwaves also cause plastic to decompose, releasing nano and microplastic particles into food. Even so-called micro-safe plastic has these problems, so it is best to never microwave anything in plastic.

What happens when you place a fruit fly in a microwave and turn it on? Nothing. The fly is smaller than the waves being produced, and they have no effect. They also don't affect microbes, which are even smaller, but hot liquids can kill them. Because of the properties of microwaves, this technique is not a good way to kill microbes in food.

Pros:

- a quick cooking method
- preserves nutrients

Cons:

- overcooking dries food and changes texture
- does not kill microbes

Slow Cooking

The slow cooker is a countertop appliance that cooks food slowly at a relatively low temperature between 170 and 280°F (77 and 138°C). Even though the temperature is lower, the closed vessel creates steam that helps destroy bacteria, making it a safe process.

The process tenderizes less expensive cuts of meat and is used to prepare complete meals in one pot. Nutrients that are lost from the food are not really lost since most recipes include the liquid in the final meal. The lower heat also helps preserve vitamins.

Pros:

- simple cooking technique
- conserves flavor

Con:

- slow process

Steaming

Steaming exposes food to hot steam without placing it directly in water. This is done in a special steamer pot or a regular pot fitted with a colander. This technique loses fewer nutrients to water.

Pros:

- preserves nutrients better than most other methods
- conserves color of vegetables better

Cons:

- requires special equipment
- used mostly for vegetables

11

Growing and Serving Quality Food

Now that you understand the basic concepts of growing and cooking food, it's time to have a look at the specifics of some common fruits and vegetables that you might grow in your garden. The focus here will be on easy-to-grow food. If you are interested in more detailed growing instructions, have a look at my YouTube channel called "Garden Fundamentals",[1] where you will find specific videos about many common vegetables.

Beans, Green (Snap Beans)

Snap beans come in a variety of cultivars and several different colors, including traditional green beans, yellow wax beans, and runner beans. These can be grouped into two basic growing styles: bush beans and pole (climbing) beans. Bush beans are smaller and start producing earlier. Provided you keep harvesting the beans, they produce for a long time. Pole beans take longer to produce the first bean, but then they produce all summer long. Beans are warm growers, so plant seed once the ground has warmed up.

Beans can be harvested when the pods are still green (or yellow, or blue) and before the seeds inside are fully ripe. Or they can be left longer and harvested as dry beans.

Growing Tricks:

- Pole beans need a structure to climb, but they will produce more food in a given space. Since they are harvested later then peas, both crops can be grown on the same trellis.
- Cover planted seed with row covers, a cloth-like material, to protect them from nibbling insects. Remove the cover once seedlings are 8 inches (20 cm) tall.
- They are usually planted directly in the garden, but they can be started inside and transplanted for an earlier harvest.
- Harvest early, when the beans still have a "snap" sound when you break them. Beans, especially runner beans, get woody very quickly. Harvest early and often.

Cooking Tricks:

- Store cold.
- Green beans contain lectins, which cause gastrointestinal problems when eaten raw. They should be cooked before eating.
- Cook as fresh as possible for best taste and don't overcook them or they get mushy. Cooked green beans should still be quite firm.

Cucumbers

Cucumbers are fairly easy to grow and they produce a good yield. They are normally started by planting seeds directly in the garden once the soil warms up. There is an old myth that recommends seeds should be planted on a hill, and you still find these instructions on seed packs. The term "hill" is an old term that used to mean "in a group." It does not mean a raised pile of soil. Unless you have a large garden where you will let the vines ramble out from the planting group, it is better to plant seeds at 4-foot intervals in a row and grow them up a trellis.

Another common myth is that you can't start them indoors because seedlings do not transfer well. If you are gentle with the seedlings, they transplant just fine and you can harvest fruit four to six weeks earlier.

The major pest of this fruit is the cucumber beetle. They are small and relentless. In small numbers they don't do much harm, except that the skin of the fruit is damaged a bit. In larger numbers they can reduce yield. Cover plants with a row cover to keep them out.

A unique characteristic of cucumbers and melons is that they have both male and female flowers. The males show up first, and are then followed by the females. You can identify females because they seem to have a growing cucumber right behind the flower even before the flower opens. Until the plant produces females, you won't get any fruit.

Growing Tricks:

- Cucumbers like lots of water, so don't let them dry out. The fruit itself is mostly water.
- Pick early while still green. Once they go yellow, the quality drops and seeds develop.
- English cucumbers are much larger to grow, so it is best to stick with American types.

Cooking Tricks:

- Pick often and use right away. Cucumbers lose moisture quickly.
- Most modern cultivars are not bitter, but the following cultivars are less bitter: Carmen, County Fair, Diva, Garden Sweet, Green Knight, Marketmore 76, Sweet Slice, Slice More, Sweet Success, Sweeter Yet, and Tasty Green.
- Cut the ends off and taste them to see if there is any bitterness. Most of the bitter compounds are found in the end of the fruit. If the ends are bitter, cut off another slice and taste again.
- This fruit does not cook or store well, but they make great pickles.

Garlic

Garlic is one of the easiest crops to grow and is available as both hardneck and softneck forms. Hardneck are more popular in cold climates, and softneck in warm areas. The term "garlic seed" is used to refer to cloves. Real seeds are actually rare on cultivated plants. The trick to planting garlic is to use the largest cloves you have. Large cloves make large bulbs the following year.

The cloves contain strong sulfur compounds that are released by enzymes when they are cut or crushed. The flavor compounds are easily lost in water and steam, but maintained in oil. Cooking in oil also adds caramelized flavors.

Growing Tricks:

- Only grow certified nematode-free garlic.
- Plant before the ground freezes.
- Don't overwater in summer.
- Remove scapes on hardnecks to get bigger bulbs.

Cooking Tricks:

- Store garlic either dry and warm, or cold in oil.
- Crushed garlic adds more taste than whole cloves.
- The best taste is obtained by cooking in oil.

Lettuce

Lettuce is available in two main types: head lettuce and leaf lettuce. Head lettuce used to be the most popular in grocery stores, but it is harder to grow. If you are a beginner, stick to leaf lettuce. It grows cool and can be started from seed either indoors or directly in the garden. Some people even start it during winter in a cold frame.

This is one vegetable that can be grown successfully in part shade. Once the weather gets warm, it bolts (i.e., goes to seed) and the leaves get bitter. There are quite a few varieties with both green and red leaves, but I think they mostly taste the same. I find oak leaf lettuce to grow and produce a good crop.

Growing Tricks:

- Start new plants in fall to get a late harvest.
- Keep well watered. This is one crop that can almost be grown sitting in water.
- For summer lettuce, grow New Zealand spinach, which is

neither a spinach nor does it come from New Zealand, but it is leafy, can be eaten like lettuce, and loves the hot summer.

Cooking Tricks:

- You can harvest a whole clump, or just cut off the outer leaves of each clump. The more you cut, the more that will grow.
- Dropping it right into water as you harvest it will keep it turgid.
- Best eaten raw and fresh.

Onion

Onions are available in a number of colors and degrees of pungency. Try different cultivars to see which you prefer. Enzymes are released when cut and they release sulfur-containing compounds that cause tearing (lachrymatory effect). Milder onions are less irritating. These flavor compounds are soluble in water and are easily lost with steam, so it best not to boil onions. They retain most of their taste when cooked in oil.

Growing Tricks:

- Growing from seed takes a long time, so it is better to plant "sets" in spring, which are baby onions.
- As they grow, the bulbs will show above ground—that is normal—just leave them.
- Harvest any time you want for green onions or small spring bulbs. The tops fall over naturally when it is time to harvest the main crop.
- Onion seed is only viable for a couple of years. It is best to buy fresh each year.

Cooking Tricks:

- Store cool, dark, and dry.
- Most tricks for preventing tearing don't work, but wearing contacts does. A sharp knife also reduces the effect because it releases fewer enzymes.
- Fry cut onions in fat or oil to retain taste and create a caramelized flavor.

Peas

Peas are cool season crops that should be planted very early. Seedlings can even take some light frost. They are available as both bush and pole types, but I find pole types produce better. There are three types of peas. Traditional shelling peas need to have the shell removed before eating. That wastes a lot of the pod and is too much work. Snow peas are harvested just as the pea starts to develop. You are eating mostly the pod and very tiny peas. Then there are Sugar Snaps, which are a hybrid between the other two. The pod is tender enough to eat, and you harvest when the peas are a good size. It is the only kind I grow.

Harvest early while the pod is still green. Once it takes on a whitish color it is too old and woody tasting.

Growing Tricks:

- Harvest with both hands. One holds the fruit stem and the other pulls off the pod. This way you won't break the tender vine.
- Harvest often so the plant keeps producing new peas. Once the weather gets hot, the plants die quickly. Try planting more in fall.
- Don't mulch right after planting to allow the sun to warm the soil. Add mulch once plants are 6 inches (15 cm) tall.

Cooking Tricks:

- Eat fresh—they don't need to be cooked.
- If you cook them, heat them for only a very short time or they get mushy.

Radish

Radishes are easy to grow, but they need to be started early and harvested before it gets too warm. Plant as soon as you can work the soil. Thin often and eat the thinnings. The common radish is red and round, but they do come in different colors, which all seem to taste the same.

Once it gets warm, radish bolts, which means they flower. Once that happens, the root is too woody for eating. Leave the plants and start harvesting the green seed pods, which taste just like radish. I like adding them to salads and fool people. They won't know where the strong radish taste is coming from. Harvest these seed pods very young, or they get woody.

Growing Tricks:

- Plant next to other crops that won't be tall until later in summer, such as carrots. The radish will be harvested before the other crop needs the space.
- Keep well watered so they grow fast.
- Replant in fall once temperatures come down.

Cooking Tricks:

- East fresh and harvest the day you need them.
- The green seed pods can be eaten fresh or stir-fried.

Raspberries

Raspberries are difficult to transport and are therefore best grown in your backyard. They are also easy to grow. There are two basic types: summer bearing and everbearing. Summer bearing are the most common. The canes growing this year do not bear fruit until the following summer. Once a cane has finished making fruit it starts to die, and needs to be removed in late summer. They produce one large harvest for a few weeks in summer.

Everbearing raspberries grow new canes this year and produce fruit on them in late summer. These same canes usually also produce some fruit the following late spring into summer. This type usually produces more fruit over a longer period of time, making it a better choice for home gardens. The old canes need to be removed once fruiting is done.

Black raspberries (*Rubus occidentalis*) grow just like the red ones except the fruit is black. There are even gold and purple colored raspberries. Blackberries (*Rubus allegheniensis*), on the other hand, are a different species. If you bought black colored berries in a grocery store, they were most likely blackberries. These can be grown similar to summer raspberries.

All of these so-called "berries" are not actually berries. They are aggregate fruits, essentially a collection of little fruits all clustered together. Strawberries are actual berries.

Growing Tricks:

- Raspberries produce lots of runners and it is best to remove most of them. Keep them contained in a single row.
- Grow raspberries in a row, with horizontal guide wires that help contain and hold up drooping canes.
- Black raspberries grow in a similar way to summer bearing red raspberries.

Cooking Tricks:

- Pick red raspberries just before they fall off the plant on their own, leaving the white center attached to the plant. Blackberries do not release from the plant, and need to be pulled off with the white center still inside the fruit.
- Both fruits make great jams and sauces, but they really are best eaten fresh.

Strawberries

Strawberries are fairly easy to grow and produce fairly well, but the real benefit to growing them is that you can get fresh strawberries. If you grow everbearing ones, you can harvest most of the summer.

There are two basic types: June bearing and everbearing. The first one produces a large crop all at one time and is used for most commercial crops. Everbearing also produces well in June, but then goes on to produce more berries for the rest of the summer.

Skip the seeds and buy starter plants in early spring. They will produce some fruit the first year, but the real harvest starts the second year. The mother plant makes runners, which lay down roots to form new plants. You can grow them in a narrow row and remove most of the runners, or grow them in a wide bed, which is my preferred method. As plants get old, remove them and also remove some baby plants if they get too crowded.

Growing Tricks:

- Keep well watered when berries are forming.
- Cover with ¼-inch hardware cloth, which keeps birds and mice out, but lets bees in for pollination.
- Mulch with straw to keep berries off the soil.
- Pick every few days to keep plants producing.

Cooking Tricks:

- Unless you plan to grow a lot, eat your harvest fresh rather than cooking them.

Tomato

Tomatoes are the most popular fruit to grow while at the same time being one of the most difficult to grow because they have several common diseases. The taste of a fresh-grown tomato is worth it.

These are tropical plants and they like warm temperatures. In cold climates, they need to be started indoors from seed and then transplanted into the garden. Or you can buy transplants in spring. They are available as miniature plants for containers, making them suitable for any size garden. They grow in two basic forms: determinate and indeterminate. Determinate are bush types that grow to a certain size and then produce their fruit. Indeterminate types grow into tall vines. This latter group produces more fruit over a longer growing season, but they do need to be staked.

Blossom end rot is a common problem that causes the blossom end of the fruit to develop a corky black area. There are dozens of myths about this problem, which has led to many DIY solutions that don't work. This is rarely a calcium deficiency. It is a watering issue. If you keep the plants evenly watered, they don't develop blossom end rot, and mulch helps a lot in this regard.[2]

Growing Tricks:

- Grow several cultivars to find the ones that grow best in your soil.
- Harvest in the breaker stage and ripen them indoors.
- Provide some shade in hot climates to keep temperatures lower, or pollination won't happen.

Cooking Tricks:

- Garden tomatoes should be eaten fresh.
- Canning at the wrong pH can lead to food poisoning, so always follow a recipe.
- Do not refrigerate. The cold temperatures result in a loss of flavor.
- Blanching makes it easy to remove skins.

Zucchini

This plant is easy to grow and produces a lot of fruit. Grow it like a cucumber plant. Start early inside and transplant once the weather is warm, or sow seed direct. Don't use hills. They form large clumps with big leaves, so space them 4 feet (120 cm) apart. They have both male and female flowers, and males form first. Once the harvest starts, the plant will produce a lot of fruit. A couple of plants is enough for a normal sized family.

Growing Tricks:

- Keep well watered, especially once fruit develops.
- Harvest when tender and a bit immature (8 inches (20 cm) long) for more flavor. They lose flavor as they get larger.

Cooking Tricks:

- Large overgrown fruit is fine for baking cakes.
- Harvest as needed—they don't store well.
- Don't overcook or they get mushy. Sauté for a couple of minutes.

Notes

Chapter 2: Understanding Nutrition

1. McCance and Widdowson, *The Composition of Foods*, 2015.
2. "Minerals: Their Functions and Sources," My Health Alberta, March 1, 2023, https://myhealth.alberta.ca/Health/Pages/conditions.aspx?hwid=ta3912.
3. "Antioxidants," Harvard T.H. Chan School of Public Health, https://www.hsph.harvard.edu/nutritionsource/antioxidants/.

Chapter 3: Food Safety—Chemicals

1. National Pesticide Information Center, http://npic.orst.edu.
2. Robert Pavlis, "The Scientific Method and Why Controls Are So Important," *Garden Myths* (blog), https://www.gardenmyths.com/scientific-method-important-controls/.
3. Bo-Han Liao et al., "Accumulation of Heavy Metals in Vegetable Species Planted in Contaminated Soils and the Health Risk Assessment," National Library of Medicine, March 4, 2016, https://www.ncbi.nlm.nih.gov/-pmc/articles/PMC4808952/.
4. Pietro Zuccarello et al., "Micro- and Nano-plastics in Edible Fruit and Vegetables. The First Diet Risks Assessment for the General Population," Science Direct, August 2020, https://www.sciencedirect.com/science/article/pii/S0013935120305703.
5. Michelle Wiesbrook, "Poisonous Plants in the Vegetable Garden," Home, Yard & Garden Pest, University of Illinois Extension, October 8, 2022, https://hyg.ipm.illinois.edu/article.php?id=1327.
6. Jon Entine, "AAAS Scientists: Consensus on GMO Safety Firmer Than For Human-Induced Climate Change," Huffpost, December 6, 2017, https://www.huffpost.com/entry/post_b_6572130.
7. "Horizontal Gene Transfer: Sweet Potato Naturally 'Genetically Modified'," Science Daily, April 21, 2015, https://www.sciencedaily.com/releases/2015/04/150421084204.htm.

8. "Genetically Modified Organisms: The Golden Rice Debate," NYU Langone Health, https://med.nyu.edu/departments-institutes/population-health/divisions-sections-centers/medical-ethics/education/high-school-bioethics-project/learning-scenarios/gmos-the-golden-rice-debate.

Chapter 4: Food Safety—Biological

1. "Burden of Foodborne Illness: Findings," Centers for Disease Control and Prevention, November 5, 2018, https://www.cdc.gov/foodborne burden/2011-foodborne-estimates.html.
2. DOE Joint Genome Institute, "JGI Plant Tissue Culture," Flickr, May 28, 2020, https://www.flickr.com/photos/doe_jgi/49946260683.
3. "Danger Zone," USDA, https://www.fsis.usda.gov/food-safety/safe-food-handling-and-preparation/food-safety-basics/danger-zone-40f-140f.
4. L. Bry, Mad Science Network, April 14, 2000, https://www.madsci.org/posts/archives/2000-04/955832137.Mi.r.html.
5. Casey Bisson, "furry-berries," Flickr, May 26, 2007, https://www.flickr.com/photos/maisonbisson/514783570.
6. John A. Painter et al., "Attribution of Foodborne Illnesses, Hospitalizations, and Deaths to Food Commodities by Using Outbreak Data, United States, 1998–2008," Emerging Infectious Diseases, Centers for Disease Control and Prevention, March 2013, https://wwwnc.cdc.gov/eid/article/19/3/11-1866_article#:~:text=We%20attributed%2046%25%20of%20illnesses,contamination%20of%20produce%20and%20poultry.
7. Robert Pavlis, "Myths About Rainwater Harvesting Systems for Gardens," *Garden Myths* (blog), https://www.gardenmyths.com/myths-rainwater-harvesting/.

Chapter 5: Nutrient Density

1. Fernando G., "File: Refractometer.jpg," Wikimedia Commons, May 19, 2006, https://commons.wikimedia.org/wiki/File:Refractometer.jpg.
2. James W. Lyne and Philip Barak, "Are Depleted Soils Causing a Reduction in the Mineral Content of Food Crops?," Dept. of Soil Science, University of Wisconsin – Madison, November 2000, http://soils.wisc.edu/facstaff/barak/poster_gallery/minneapolis2000a/.
3. Donald R. Davis et al., "Changes in USDA Food Composition Data for 43 Garden Crops, 1950 to 1999," National Library of Medicine, December 2004, https://www.ncbi.nlm.nih.gov/pubmed/15637215.
4. Robin J. Marles, "Mineral Nutrient Composition of Vegetables, Fruits and Grains," Science Direct, March 2017, https://www.sciencedirect.com/science/article/pii/S0889157516302113?via%3Dihub.

Chapter 6: The Flavor of Food

1. G. M. Sapers et al., "Tomato Acidity and the Safety of Home Canned Tomatoes," *HortScience*, June 1977, https://journals.ashs.org/hortsci/view/journals/hortsci/12/3/article-p204.xml.
2. G. M. Sapers et al., "Tomato Acidity."
3. Anuschka Heeb et al., "Impact of Organic and Inorganic Fertilizers on Yield, Taste, and Nutritional Quality of Tomatoes," Wiley Online Library, August 18, 2006, https://onlinelibrary.wiley.com/doi/abs/10.1002/jpln.200520553.
4. F. J. McArdle et al., "Pesticides and Food Flavor, Influence of Herbicides on Flavor of Processed Fruits and Vegetables," ACS Publications, May 1, 1961, https://pubs.acs.org/doi/10.1021/jf60115a016.

Chapter 7: Growing Great Food

1. Robert Pavlis, "Vegetable Gardening Master Class," Garden Fundamentals, February 12, 2022, YouTube video, https://youtu.be/-8FhheT3TlI.
2. "'Organic' Food Labels Create Perception of Healthier Fare," Cornell Chronicle, April 26, 2011, https://news.cornell.edu/stories/2011/04/organic-food-label-imparts-health-halo-study-finds.
3. Michelle Brandt, "Little Evidence of Health Benefits from Organic Foods, Study Finds," Stanford Medicine, September 3, 2012, https://med.stanford.edu/news/all-news/2012/09/little-evidence-of-health-benefits-from-organic-foods-study-finds.html.
4. Mary Jane Brown et al., "Antibiotics in Your Food: Should You Be Concerned?," Healthline, June 23, 2023, https://www.healthline.com/nutrition/antibiotics-in-your-food#TOC_TITLE_HDR_3.
5. Luke Denne and Tiffany Foxcroft, "'People Are Being Duped': CBC Exposes Homegrown Lies at Farmers Markets," CBC Marketplace, November 30, 2017, https://www.cbc.ca/news/business/farmers-markets-lies-marketplace-1.4306231.
6. Brie Dyas, "Is the Produce at the Farmers Market Local? Turns Out, Not Always," Huffpost, June 27, 2018, https://www.huffpost.com/entry/farmers-market-local-produce_n_5b315478e4b0b5e692f0a414.
7. Chenchen Ren et al,. "The Impact of Farm Size on Agricultural Sustainability," Science Direct, May 20, 2019, https://www.sciencedirect.com/science/article/abs/pii/S0959652619305402#:~:text=Farm%20size%20plays%20a%20critical,excessive%20use%20of%20mineral%20fertilizers.
8. Fábio Cunha Coelho et al, "Local Food: Benefits and Failings due to Modern Agriculture," Scielo Brazil, January–February 2018, https://www.scielo.br/j/sa/a/DNPPhm8L8RD9zGQtzrjCwhf/?lang=en&stop=next&format=html.

Chapter 8: Handling and Storing Food

1. Robert Pavlis, "7 Best Ways to Wash Fruits and Vegetables," *Garden Myths* (blog), https://www.gardenmyths.com/wash-fruits-vegetables/.
2. Paul Dawson and Brian Sheldon, *Did You Just Eat That?* W.W. Norton & Company, November 6, 2018.
3. "Ethylene in Fruits and Vegetables," USD Community Health, https://ucsdcommunityhealth.org/wp-content/uploads/2017/09/ethylene.pdf.
4. Ron Goldy, "All Fruit and Vegetables Are Not Created Equal When It Comes to Proper Storage Conditions," MSU Extension, Michigan State University, January 23, 2019, https://www.canr.msu.edu/news/all-fruit-and-vegetables-are-not-created-equal-when-it-comes-to-proper-storage-conditions.
5. "Storing Fresh Fruits and Vegetables for Best Flavor," Extension Purdue, https://extension.purdue.edu/foodlink/includes/pubs/Storing%20Fruits%20and%20Veggies.pdf.

Chapter 9: Preserving Food

1. "Vegetable Blanching Directions and Times for Home Freezer Storage," University of Minnesota Extension, 2023, https://extension.umn.edu/preserving-and-preparing/vegetable-blanching-directions-and-times-home-freezer-storage.
2. Jonathunder, "File:BallBlue.jpg," Wikimedia Commons, April 10, 2011, https://commons.wikimedia.org/wiki/File:BallBlue.jpg.
3. "Canning Quick Reference Chart," University of Minnesota Extension, 2021, https://extension.umn.edu/preserving-and-preparing/canning-quick-reference-chart.
4. Barbara Willenberg, "How to Use Dehydrated Foods," Extension University of Missouri, May 2018, https://extension.missouri.edu/publications/gh1564#:~:text=When%20using%20dehydrated%20products%20you,the%20desired%20volume%20is%20restored.
5. Kevin Whelan et al., "Fermented Foods: Definitions and Characteristics, Impact on the Gut Microbiota and Effects on Gastrointestinal Health and Disease," National Library of Medicine, August 5, 2019, https://www.ncbi.nlm.nih.gov/pmc/articles/PMC6723656/.
6. Ronald B. Pegg et al., "Selected Nutrient Analyses of Fresh, Fresh-Stored, and Frozen Fruits and Vegetables," Science Direct, June 2017, https://www.sciencedirect.com/science/article/abs/pii/S0889157517300418.
7. "Cold Food Storage Chart," Food Safety.gov, September 19, 2023, https://www.foodsafety.gov/food-safety-charts/cold-food-storage-charts.

8. "How to Pasteurize Milk at Home," My Health Alberta, February 24, 2021, https://myhealth.alberta.ca/Alberta/Pages/how-to-pasteurize-milk.aspx#:~:text=Keep%20the%20milk%20at%20the,have%20to%20start%20timing%20again.

Chapter 10: Cooking Food

1. Devon Wagner, "How to Reduce Arsenic in Rice, and Why It Matters," Ohio State Health & Discovery, January 18, 2023, https://health.osu.edu/wellness/exercise-and-nutrition/how-to-reduce-arsenic-in-rice.
2. https://ifst.onlinelibrary.wiley.com/doi/10.1111/jfpp.16590.
3. Hoonjeong Kwon et al., "Effect of Cooking Method on the Concentrations of Volatile N-nitrosamines in Various Food Products," Institute of Food Science & Technology, July 2022, https://inspection.canada.ca/food-safety-for-industry/food-chemistry-and-microbiology/food-safety-testing-reports-and-journal-articles/final-report/eng/1578610274684/1578610437111.
4. Robert Pavlis, "Will Oxalic Acid in Rhubarb Leaves Harm You?," *Garden Myths* (blog), https://www.gardenmyths.com/oxalic-acid-rhubarb-leaves-harm-you/.

Chapter 11: Growing and Serving Quality Food

1. Robert Pavlis, "Garden Fundamentals Introduction," Garden Fundamentals, 2018 YouTube video, http://www.youtube.com/Gardenfundamentals1.
2. Robert Pavlis, "Blossom End Rot," *Garden Myths* (blog), https://www.gardenmyths.com/blossom-end-rot/.

Index

Page numbers in *italics* indicate figures and tables.

A

acetic acid, 36
ACQ treated wood, 50
acrylamide, 167–168
acute toxicity, 35
aerobic bacteria, 66
agriculture, farm size, 117–118
Agrobacterium, 54–55
air exclusion, to preserve, 137
alcoholic fermentation, 145
allelopathy, 50, 52–53
allergies, 56–57
alum, 155
aluminum, 168
aluminum sulfate, 41
amino acids, 14–15
anaerobic bacteria, 66
animal food products, antibiotics in, 116–117
anthocyanin, 54
antibiotics, 23, 116–117
antibodies, 14
antinutrients, 12
antioxidants, 27–28
appearance of food, 90–91
Appert, Nicholas, 137
appetite, 4
apples, 37, 69–70, 169
Arctic apple, 69–70
aroma, 91
arsenic, 41, 43, 49–50
artificial flavors, 95
asbestos, 35, 36
ascorbic acid (vitamin C), 22, 36

B

B vitamins, 23
bacteria, about, 60
  See also microbes
baking, 173
bananas, 34, 131
barbecuing, 176, 178
Barker, Allen V., 83–84
beans, dried, 18, 144, 169
beans, green, 102, 118, 169, 181–182
beer, 149
beets, 165–166
bell peppers, 121
berries, 128–129, 161
"best by" dates, 69
beta-carotene, 55
bioavailability, enhancement of, 12
biodensity. *See* nutrient density
biofilm, 126
biological food safety, about, 59–60
  See also foodborne illnesses
bisphenol A (BPA), 46, 47
bitter taste, 91–93, 100
blanching, 136, 137, 178
bleach, 172
blood pressure, 31
blueberries, 27
boiling, 136, 173–174
botulism, 138, 153
bound water, 65
bread, 147, 149
Brix scale, 77–80
broccoli, 100, 103
broiling, 176, 178
bromelain, 16

brown sugar, 19
Burpee, 109
bush beans, 118

C
cabbage, 83–84, 103
cadmium, 42, 43
calcium, 11–12, 24, 83
calories, 13–14
Campylobacter, 60
cancer, 26, 165
canning, 137–141, *140*
caramelization, 161–162
carbohydrates, 17–19
carotenoids, 162–163
carrots, 43, 99, 102, 105, 119
cassava, 169
cauliflower, 103
cedar, for raised beds, 50
cereals, 12
chemical pesticides, 40
chemicals
  detection of, 36–37
  microplastics, 51
  plastics, 45–48, 179
  in raised bed materials, 48–50
  toxicity, 35–36
  types of, 33–35
  See also pesticides
chilling injury, 131
chlorophyll, 162–163
chocolate, 43
cholecalciferol (vitamin D), 22
cholesterol, 31
chromium, 41
chronic toxicity, 35, 36
clay soil, 99
climacteric fruit, 122
climate, effect on nutrients, 30–31, 86–87
Clostridium botulinum, 138, 153
complete protein sources, 16–17
compost, 74
concrete blocks, for raised beds, 49
containers, 45–47, 88
cooking
  compounds created by, 165–168
  effect on flavor, 161–164
  effect on nutrients, 164–165
  foods that require, 169–170, 172
  methods, 172–180
  reasons to, 159–160
copper, 24, 41, 50, 82
copper sulfate, 40, 114–115
corrugated metal, for raised beds, 50–51
COVID vaccine, 55
cucumbers, 100, 102, 182–183
cultivar, definition, 107
cultivar selection, 30, 101, 106–107
cutting produce, effect on flavor, 103
cyanide, 35–36, 91

D
daffodils, 52
"danger zone" temperature range, 67, *67*
days to maturity, 107–108, 118
DDT, 38
dehydration, 142–143, 144, *145*
detox diets, 32
diet, healthy, 4
diets, 31, 32
digestibility, of food, 159–160
digestion process, 3–4
diphenylamine, 37
Dirty Dozen, 37–38
drinks, fermented, *148*
dry heat cooking, 172
drying foods, 65
drying seeds, 144

E
E. coli, 60, 66, 67
eating, reasons for, 3–4
eggs, 30, 31, 169
elderberry, 170
Enterohemorrhagic *E. coli*, 60
Environmental Working Group (EWG), 37–38
enzymatic browning, 69–70
enzymes, 14, 15–16
essential amino acids, 14–15, 16–17
ethylene gas, 122–124

F
F1 hybrid, 110
facultative anaerobes, 66
farm size, 117–118
fats and oils
about, 19–20
cooking in, 175
effect of heating, 177
myths about, 31
smoke point, *176*
fatty acids, 20
fermentation, 144–147, *148*, 149–150, *154*
fertilizer, 100, 116
fiber, 18–19
fiddleheads, 170
five-second rule, 129
flavonoids, 162–163
flavor
definition, 89–90
effect of cooking, 160, 161–164
factors affecting, 90–94, 96–98
in homegrown food, 98–103, 105–106
nutrition and, 94–96
Flavor Extract Manufacturers Association (FEMA), 89
fluoride, 24, 35
folic acid (vitamin B9), 23
food
antibiotics in, 116–117
buying safe food, 70
detecting microbe contamination, 68
fermented, *148*
local food, 117–118
nutrient density, 75–76, 82–83
pathogen myths and, 71–74
taste of purchased, 96
food allergies, 56–57
Food and Drug Administration (FDA), 95
food intolerances, 56–57
food manufacturing companies, standards, 5
food poisoning. *See* foodborne illnesses
food quality, 5, 6, 7–9, 90–91
food safe plastics, 46–47, *46*
food safety
about, 33
"best by" dates, 69
biological, 59–60
detecting microbe contamination, 68
effect of cooking, 160–161
intrinsic factors for microbe growth, 63
pathogen myths and, 71–74
when purchasing, 70
See also chemicals; foodborne illnesses
food science, 3, 9–10
foodborne illnesses
about, 59–60
causes of, 60–61
identifying contamination, 68
prevention, 71–74
produce and, 70–71
types of, 61–62
free radicals, 27–28
freeze drying, 143–144
freezer burn, 151
freezing, 73, 136, 150–153, *152*
fructose, 17–18, *18*
fruit
browning, 69–70
canning times, *140*
development stages, 120
effect of cooking, 161
fermentation, 149–150
harvest, 121–122
juice pasteurization, 153
preferred storage temperatures, *132–133*
ripening, 102, 122–124
frying, 175
fungi, 61

G
gardeners, advice from, 106
gardens, pathogens in, 73–74
garlic, 103, 153, 183–184
garlic mustard (*Alliaria petiolate*), 53

gelatin salad, 16
genetics, effect on nutrients, 86, 88
gloves, 126
glucose, 17, *18*
glyphosate (Roundup), 33, 36, 37
GMO (genetically modified organism)
  food, 53–56, 85
  seeds, 109, 111
grain, 84
green beans, 102, 118, 169, 181–182
grilling, 176, 178
growing
  effect on flavor, 98–101
  evaluating nutrition, 77
  factors affecting nutrients, 6–7, 29–31, 85–86
  factors affecting quality, 7–9
  focus on quantity, 105–106
growing season, extension of, 118–120
growth hormones, 116
gut microbiome, 146, 147

H
handling food, 125–129
hands, importance of washing, 126
harvest, 6, 101–102, 108, 118–122
heart disease, 31, 32
heat. *See* temperature
heavy metals, 41–45
The Heirloom Gardener, 109
heirloom seeds, 108–109, 111–114
hepatitis A, 60, 71, 73
heterocyclic amines (HCAs), 167, 176
home grown. *See* growing
home remedies, pesticides, 40
honey, 32
honeydew melons, 131
hot compost, 74
human nutrients, plant nutrients vs, 12–13
humidity, food storage and, 66, 130–131
hybrid seeds, 110
hyperaccumulators, 42

I
imported food, nutrition level, 6
infection, 62
intoxication, 61–62
iron, 12, 24
irradiation, 157

J
juglone, 52–53
juice pasteurization, 153

K
kale, 100
kefir, 147, *148*
Klee Lab, 109, 112

L
lactic acid fermentation, 145
Lamborn, Calvin, 112
LD50 (lethal dose + 50%), 35–36
lead, 42, 43, 88
lectins, 169
legumes, 12, 18, 57
lettuce
  growing and cooking tips, 184–185
  growing season, 118
  heavy metal absorption, 43
  mineral levels, 83, 84
  selecting cultivars, 106–107
leucine, 15
lima beans, 170
local food, 6–7, 117–118
lyophilization, 143–144

M
Maillard reaction, 162
manure, 72
Mason, John, 137
maturity dates, 107–108, 118
meat, 32, *142*
melons, 100
menaquinone (vitamin K), 23
mercury, 41
messenger proteins, 14
Mexican fireweed (*Bassia scoparia*), 53

microbes
- effect of freeze drying, 143
- effect of freezing, 151
- foodborne illness myths, 71–74
- foodborne illnesses, 59–60, 61–62
- growth environment, 63–68
- killing by cooking myths, 172
- sources of on produce, 126
- transference to food, 129
- types of, 60–61

microplastics, 51
microwave ovens, 73, 178–179
milk pasteurization, 153
milkweed, 38
minerals
- about, 25
- effect of cooking, 164
- function in humans, *24*
- soil fertility and, 81–82
- taste and, 97
- when pressure canning, 141

mint, 89
moist heat cooking, 172
moisture content, 28–29, *28*
moisture reduction, 137
molasses, 19
mold, 61, 65, 73
monarch butterflies, 38
mouthfeel, 93–94
mulch, 48, 50, 87

N

National Cancer Institute, 75
National Institute of Health, 11
natural chemicals, 34
natural flavors, 95
natural pesticides, 38–40, *39*
New Zealand spinach, 118–119
nicotine, 33, 34
nightshade family, 34
nitrates, 165–166
nitrogen, 99
nitrosamines, 166–167
non-climacteric fruit, 122
nontasters, 92
norovirus, 60
nutrient density
- definition, 75–76
- factors affecting, 80–83, 86–88
- measurement of, 76–80
- research, 83–86

nutrient-rich food index (NRF), 75
nutrients
- effect of cooking, 164–165
- effect of freezing, 152
- flavor and, 94–96
- growing factors affecting, 29–31
- in homegrown food, 6, 105
- human vs plant, 12–13
- in organic foods, 115–116
- in water from boiling foods, 174

nutrition
- definition, 11
- measurement of, 6–7, 8
- scientist recommendations, 9–10

O

odors, 91, 102–103
oil packing, 153
oils. *See* fats and oils
olive oil, 177
onions, 43, 99, 103, 119, 185
open-pollinated, 110
organic, heirloom vs, 111
organic food
- certification, 114–115
- chemical exposure, 116–117
- grown in plastic containers, 47
- pathogens in, 72
- pesticides used, 40

organic matter, 88, 99
osmosis, 136, 161
oxalic acid, 12, 25, 171
oxygen, microbe growth and, 66

P

paint, 42, 43, 88
papaya, 55
parasites, 61
Parker, M. C., 112
pasta water, 174
Pasteur, Louis, 137

pasteurization, 153
pathogens. *See* microbes
peanuts, 57
peas, 18, 52, 112, 122, 186
peeling produce, 71–72
pesticides
  amount ingested, 39
  contaminated fruits and vegetables, 37–38
  effect on flavor, 100
  heavy metals in, 42
  natural, 38–40, 116
  in organic farming, 114–115
  in organic foods, 40
  pathogens and, 72
  washing off, 127–128
PETE plastic, 47
pH, 64–65, 97
phthalates, 45–46
phylloquinone (vitamin K), 23
phytic acid, 12, 25
Phytochemical Index (PI), 26
phytonutrients, 25–27, 96
phytoremediation, 42
pickling, 154–156, *154*
pigmentation loss, in cooking, 162–163
pineapple, 16
plant nutrients, human nutrients vs, 12–13
plant pots, 45–47, 88
plant protein, 17
plants, chemicals in, 38–40, 42–43, 51–52, 116
plastic mulch, 48
plasticizers, 45–46
plastics, 45–48, 51, 179
poaching, 173–174
poison hemlock (*Conium maculatum*), 52
poisoning, 35
pole beans, 118
pollination, 110, 111, 113
polycyclic aromatic hydrocarbons (PAHs), 167, 176
polyphenol oxidase, 69–70
polypropylene, 47
polysaccharides, 18, 163–164
potatoes
  effect of cooking, 167–168
  nutrients, 32
  toxins, 35, 52, 169, 170, 172
preservation techniques
  methods, 137, 139–147, 149–157
  nutrient level and, 7, 32
  purpose of, 135
  scientific principles used, 136–137
preservatives, 136
pressure canning, 139–141
pressure-treated wood, 41, 44, 49–50
produce
  foodborne illnesses, 70–71
  pathogens and, 71–72
  store-bought flavor, 96
  washing, 125, 126–128
protein, 12–15, *15*, 16–17, 163
PVC (polyvinyl chloride), 47
pyrethrin, 33

Q
quantity, focus in growing, 105–106

R
radishes, 102, 103, 118, 119, 186–187
raffinose, 18
rain barrels, 74
raised beds, 8, 48–51, 88
raspberries, 187–188
red meat, 32
refractometers, 77–78
refrigerators, 131
rehydration, 144, *145*
relative humidity, 130–131
retinol (vitamin A), 21–22, 55
rhubarb, 12, 171
rice, 43, 55
rice water, 174
ricin, 33, 40
ringspot virus disease, 55
ripeness, 102, 130–132
roads, 44
roasting, 173

S

safety. *See* chemicals; food safety
safety standards, for food manufacturing, 5
salt, 99
salting, to preserve, 156
salty taste, 91–93
sandy soil, 99
saturated fats, 20, 31
sautéeing, 175
scurvy, 22
seed catalogs, 106
seeds
 cultivar selection, 30, 106–107
 days to maturity, 107–108
 drying, 144
 heirloom, 108–109, 111–114
 hybrid, 110
Séralini, Gilles-Eric, 55
shade, impact on plant growth, 87
simmering, 173–174
slow cookers, 179
smell, 89–90
smoke point, *176*, 177
snap beans, 102, 118, 169, 181–182
soap, 71, 126
sodium, 24, 31, 99
sodium fluoride, 35
soil
 effect of fertility, 80–82, 99
 effect on nutrients, 30–31, 86, 87–88
 heavy metal contamination, 43–45
 pathogens in, 73–74
soil analysis, 88
solanine, 34, 35, 170, 172
sour taste, 91–93, 95
Spain, glyphosate testing, 37
spinach, 12, 43
spoilage, 68, 71
sprouts, 169
standards, for food manufacturing, 5
steaming, 180
stir-frying, 175
storage
 effect on flavor, 102–103, 130–132
 effect on nutrients, 85
 extrinsic factors for microbe growth, 63
 of frozen food, *152*
 preferred temperatures, *132–133*
strawberries, 188–189
structural proteins, 14
succession planting, 118
sugar (sucrose), 17–18, *18*, 19, 32, 65
Sugar Snap peas, 112
sulfur, 24, 99
sunflowers, 42–43, 53, 144
sunlight, 47, 87
superfoods, 27
supertasters, 92
sweet peas, 52
sweet potatoes, 54–55, 169
sweet taste, 91–93, 95
synthetic chemicals, 34
synthetic pesticides, 39, *39*

T

table sugar (sucrose), 17–18, *18*, 19, 32, 65
Tanksley, Steven, 114
taste, 89, 91–93, 112–113, 115
 See also flavor
taste buds, 90, 91–93
taste preferences, 4
temperature
 carcinogen production, 141
 effect on flavor, 100–101
 effect on plastics, 47
 food storage and, 130, 131, 136
 freezing to destroy pathogens, 73
 microbe growth and, 66–68
test kits, 88
texture of food, 93–94
tocopherol (vitamin E), 22–23
tomatine, 34–35
tomatoes
 days to maturity, *108*
 GMO seeds, 54
 growing and cooking tips, 189–190
 heirlooms, 111–112
 low acid, 30, 97–98
 nutrient levels, 84

- ripening, 102, 123
- toxins, 34–35

tongue map, 92–93
toxic plants, 51–52
toxicoinfection, 62
toxins, 32, 51–52, 165–168
transpiration, 130
transport proteins, 14
transportation of food, 118
treated wood, 41, 44, 49–50
triglycerides, 19–20
tryptophan, 15

U

umami, 92, 95
unbound water, 65
unsaturated fats, 20
untreated wood, for raised beds, 49
US Department of Agriculture, 75
UV light, effect on plastics, 47

V

vacuum sealing, 66, 156
variety, definition, 107
vegetables
- canning times, *140*
- dehydration temperatures, *142*
- heavy metal absorption, 44–45
- preferred storage temperatures, *132–133*
- raw vs cooked, 164–165
- water from boiling, 174

vinegar, 33, 36
viruses, 60
- *See also* microbes

vitamin A (retinol), 21–22, 55
vitamin B, 23
vitamin B9 (folic acid), 23
vitamin C (ascorbic acid), 22, 36
vitamin D (cholecalciferol), 22
vitamin E (tocopherol), 22–23
vitamin K (phylloquinone, menaquinone), 23
vitamins, 20–21, 141, 164

W

Wagner, Tom, 111
walnut trees, 52–53
washing, 125–129
water
- about, 28
- effect on flavor, 99–100
- glyphosate testing in Spain, 37
- impact on plant growth, 87
- microbe growth and, 65
- moisture content of foods, 28
- pathogens in, 73–74
- requirements for intake, 29

water bath canning, 139
wine, 149–150
wood, for raised beds, 41, 44, 49–50

Y

yeast
- about, 61
- fermented foods, 145, 147, 149–150
- water requirements, 65

Z

zucchini, 190

About the Author

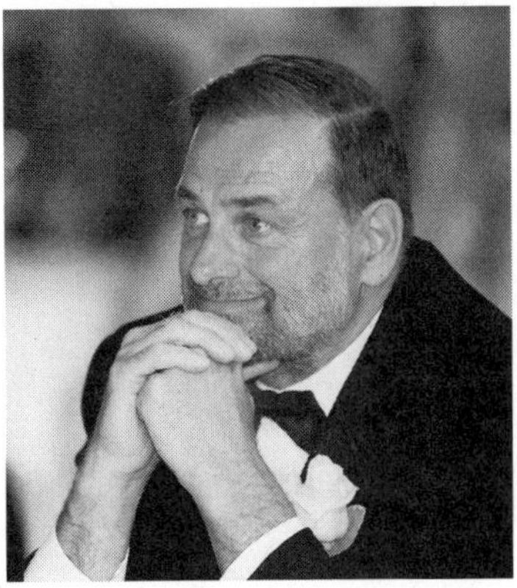

Robert Pavlis, a Master Gardener with over 45 years of gardening experience, is owner and developer of Aspen Grove Gardens, a six-acre botanical garden featuring 3,000 varieties of plants. A popular and well-respected speaker and teacher, Robert has published articles in *Mother Earth News*, *Ontario Gardening* magazine, a monthly plant of the month column for the Ontario Rock Garden Society website, and local newspapers. He is also the author of one widely read blog: GardenMyths.com, which explodes common gardening myths and provides gardening and garden design information. Robert also has a gardening YouTube channel called Garden Fundamentals.

Connect with Robert Pavlis

You can connect with me through social media by leaving comments at one of the following:

- http://www.gardenmyths.com
- http://www.youtube.com/Gardenfundamentals1

The best way to reach me directly is through my Facebook Group: https://www.facebook.com/groups/GardenFundamentals, where I answer questions on a daily basis.

Also by the Author

Microbe Science for Gardeners

Microscopic organisms are as important to plant growth as water and light. *Microbe Science for Gardeners* highlights the essential role of microbes in plant biosystems and soil health, provides practical how-to gardening advice for enhancing plant microbiomes, and debunks common gardening myths.

This accessible guide goes beyond soil biology to examine the crucial role of microorganisms in cultivating a productive garden. Coverage includes:

- the vital interrelationships in microbe populations and between microbes and plants
- understanding microbes such as bacteria, yeast, mycorrhizal fungi, and protozoa, both in the rhizosphere and above ground
- scientific breakthroughs about microbes that live in the leaves and roots of plants, forming symbiotic relationships

- how practices such as tilling, crop rotation, and mulching affect the microbe community
- how the savvy gardener can influence microbial colonies to encourage beneficial organisms while discouraging those that cause disease or other undesirable effects
- an objective, common-sense analysis of recently popularized practices such as controlling fungal-to-bacterial ratios and applying biostimulants, compost tea, or plant probiotics
- prevention and cures for dozens of bacterial, viral, and fungal plant diseases.

Whether you're a home gardener, market gardener, or micro-farmer, *Microbe Science for Gardeners* will help you leverage the incredible power of the mighty microbe to grow healthy, strong, thriving plants.

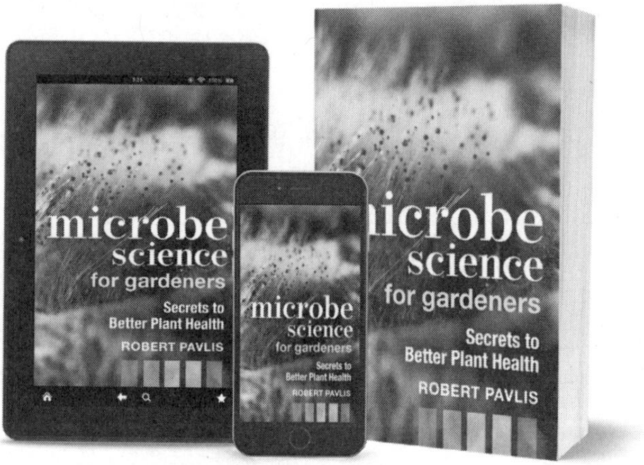

Compost Science for Gardeners

With breathtaking clarity, *Compost Science for Gardeners* demystifies composting practices and helps readers determine the best technique for their unique situation. This comprehensive science-based book is your key to building healthier soil and growing better plants.

Using plain language and easy-to-follow instructions, this essential resource distills and blends the latest scientific research with the author's many decades of knowledge and experience into manageable form, debunking a host of common gardening myths along the way. Learn about:

- the role of composting in the ecological cycle
- compostable materials to incorporate and those to avoid
- browns and greens vs the carbon-to-nitrogen ratio
- the full range of composting methods, including cold and hot composting; composting in piles, bins, and tumblers; and pit and trench composting
- keyhole gardening, food digesters, vermicomposting, bokashi, eco-enzyme fermentation, and more
- the relative merits and impact on the environment of each composting technique
- using finished compost to improve soil health

Anyone can compost. Whether you are a balcony or backyard gardener, market gardener, small-scale farmer, or homesteader, or even if you are simply looking for a way to keep organic matter out of the landfill, this book will show you how to do it simply, safely, and sensibly.

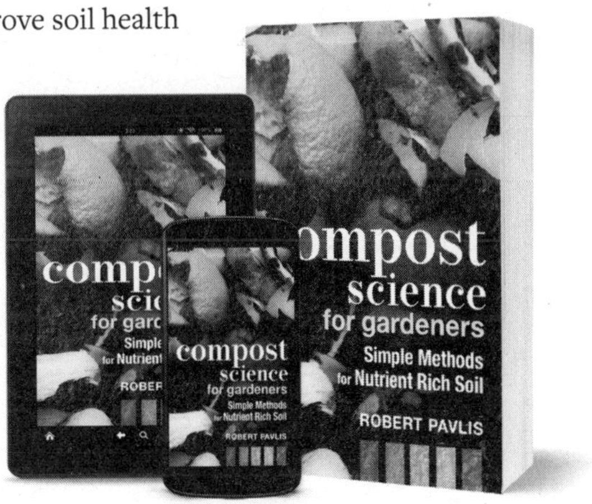

Plant Science for Gardeners

Plant Science for Gardeners empowers growers to analyze common problems, find solutions, and make better decisions in the garden for optimal plant health and productivity.

By understanding the basic biology of how plants grow, you can become a thinking gardener with the confidence to problem solve for optimized plant health and productivity. Learn the science and ditch the rules! Coverage includes:

- the biology of roots, stems, leaves, and flowers
- understanding how plants function as whole organisms
- the role of nutrients and inputs
- vegetables, flowers, grasses, and trees and shrubs
- propagation and genetics
- sidebars that explode common gardening myths
- tips for evaluating plant problems and finding solutions.

Whether you're a home gardener, micro-farmer, market gardener, or homesteader, this entertaining and accessible guide shortens the learning curve and gives you the knowledge to succeed no matter where you live.

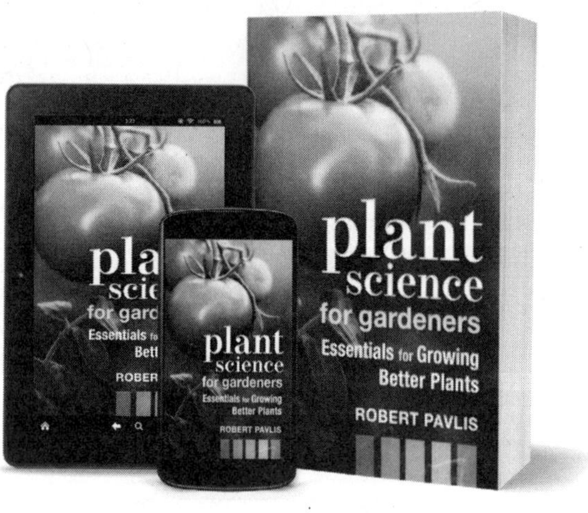

Soil Science for Gardeners

Robert Pavlis, a gardener for over four decades, debunks common soil myths, explores the rhizosphere, and provides a personalized soil fertility improvement program in this three-part popular science guidebook. Coverage includes:

- soil biology and chemistry and how plants and soil interact
- common soil health problems, including analyzing soil's fertility and plant nutrients
- the creation of a personalized plan for improving your soil fertility, including setting priorities and goals in a cost-effective, realistic time frame.
- creating the optimal conditions for nature to do the heavy lifting of building soil fertility

Written for the home gardener, market gardener, and micro-farmer, *Soil Science for Gardeners* is packed with information to help you grow thriving plants.

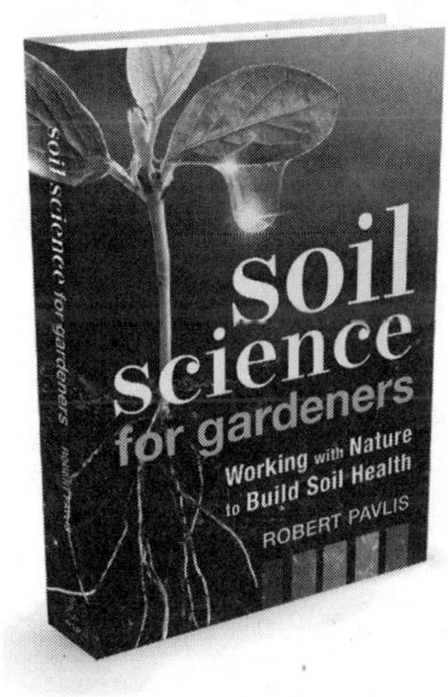

Garden Myths

If you enjoyed this book you may also like Robert's other books, *Garden Myths Book 1* and *Garden Myths Book 2*. Each one examines over 120 horticultural urban legends.

Turning wisdom on its head, Robert Pavlis dives deep into traditional garden advice and debunks the myths and misconceptions that abound. He asks critical questions and uses science-based information to understand plants and their environment. Armed with the truth, Robert then turns this knowledge into easy-to-follow advice. Details about the book can be found at http://www.gardenmyths.com/garden-myths-book-1/. They are available from Amazon, and other online outlets.

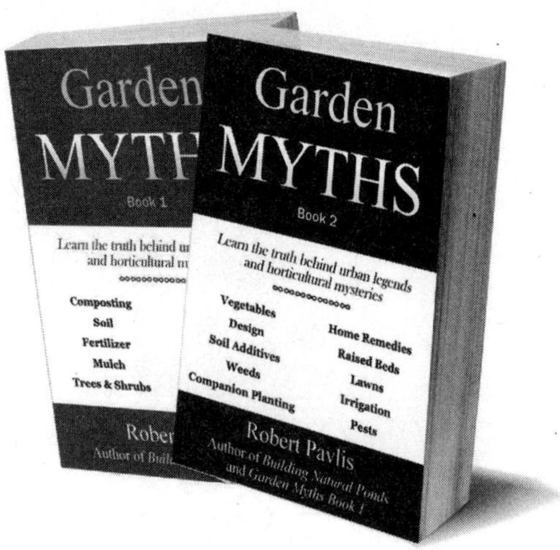

Building Natural Ponds

Building Natural Ponds is the first step-by-step guide to designing and building natural ponds that use no pumps, filters, chemicals, or electricity and mimic native ponds in both aesthetics and functionality. Highly illustrated with how-to drawings and photographs.

For more information and ordering details, visit: www.BuildingNaturalPonds.com

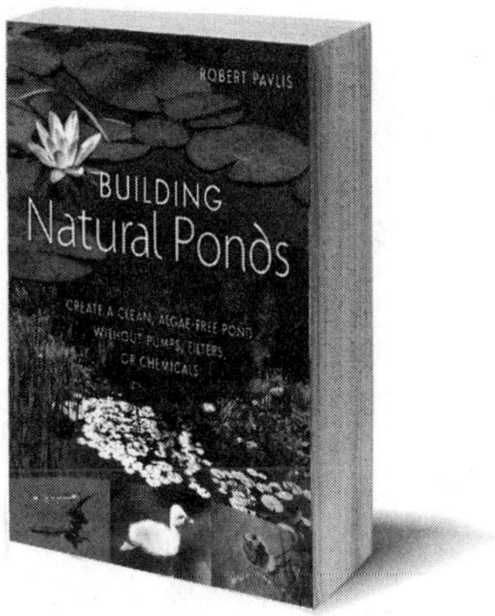

ABOUT NEW SOCIETY PUBLISHERS

New Society Publishers is an activist, solutions-oriented publisher focused on publishing books to build a more just and sustainable future. Our books offer tips, tools, and insights from leading experts in a wide range of areas.

We're proud to hold to the highest environmental and social standards of any publisher in North America. When you buy New Society books, you are part of the solution!

At New Society Publishers, we care deeply about *what* we publish—but also about *how* we do business.

- This book is printed on 100% **post-consumer recycled paper**, processed chlorine-free, with low-VOC vegetable-based inks (since 2002)
- Our corporate structure is an innovative employee shareholder agreement, so we're one-third employee-owned (since 2015)
- We've created a Statement of Ethics (2021). The intent of this Statement is to act as a framework to guide our actions and facilitate feedback for continuous improvement of our work
- We're carbon-neutral (since 2006)
- We're certified as a B Corporation (since 2016)
- We're Signatories to the UN's Sustainable Development Goals (SDG) Publishers Compact (2020–2030, the Decade of Action)

To download our full catalog, sign up for our quarterly newsletter, and to learn more about New Society Publishers, please visit newsociety.com.

ENVIRONMENTAL BENEFITS STATEMENT

New Society Publishers saved the following resources by printing the pages of this book on chlorine free paper made with 100% post-consumer waste.

TREES	WATER	ENERGY	SOLID WASTE	GREENHOUSE GASES
36 FULLY GROWN	2,900 GALLONS	15 MILLION BTUs	120 POUNDS	15,800 POUNDS

Environmental impact estimates were made using the Environmental Paper Network Paper Calculator 4.0. For more information visit www.papercalculator.org

Certified B Corporation

new society PUBLISHERS www.newsociety.com

FSC www.fsc.org MIX Paper | Supporting responsible forestry FSC® C016245

SDG PUBLISHERS COMPACT